# UROGENITAL INFECTIONS

## New Developments in Laboratory Diagnosis and Treatment

# ADVANCES IN EXPERIMENTAL MEDICINE AND BIOLOGY



## Recent Volumes in this Series

Volume 218
CORONAVIRUSES
Edited by Michael M. C. Lai and Stephen A. Stohlman

Volume 219
REGULATION OF OVARIAN AND TESTICULAR FUNCTION
Edite by Virendra B. Mahesh, Dharam S. Dhindsa, Everett Anderson, and Satya P. Kalra

Volume 220
CONTINUOUS TRANSCUTANEOUS MONITORING
Edited by Albert Huch, Renate Huch, and Gosta Rooth

Volume 221
MOLECULAR MECHANISMS OF NEURONAL RESPONSIVENESS
Edited by Yigal H. Ehrlich, Robert H. Lenox, Elizabeth Kornecki, and William O. Berry

Volume 222
OXYGEN TRANSPORT TO TISSUE X
Edited by Masaji Mochizuki, Carl R. Honig, Tomiyasu Koyama, Thomas K. Goldstick, and Duane F. Bruley

Volume 223
UREMIC TOXINS
Edited by Severin Ringoir, Raymond Vanholder, and Shaul G. Massry

Volume 224
UROGENITAL INFECTIONS: New Developments in Laboratory Diagnosis and Treatment
Edited by Amedeo Bondi, Donald D. Stieritz, Joseph M. Campos, and Linda Ann Miller

Volume 225
IMMUNOBIOLOGY OF PROTEINS AND PEPTIDES IV: T-CELL RECOGNITION AND ANTIGEN PRESENTATION
Edited by M. Zouhair Atassi

# UROGENITAL INFECTIONS

## New Developments in Laboratory Diagnosis and Treatment

Edited by

**Amedeo Bondi** and
**Donald D. Stieritz**
Hahnemann University
Philadelphia, Pennsylvania

**Joseph M. Campos**
Children's Hospital
National Medical Center
Washington, D.C.

and

**Linda Ann Miller**
Holy Redeemer Hospital and Medical Center
Meadowbrook, Pennsylvania

PLENUM PRESS • NEW YORK AND LONDON

Library of Congress Cataloging in Publication Data

Eastern Pennsylvania Branch of the American Society for Microbiology Symposium on Urogenital Infections: New Developments in Laboratory Diagnosis and Treatment (1984: Philadelphia, Pa.)
Urogenital infections.

(Advances in experimental medicine and biology; v. 224)
"Based on the proceedings of the Eastern Pennsylvania Branch of the American Society for Microbiology Symposium on Urogenital Infections: New Developments in Laboratory Diagnosis and Treatment, held November 15-16, 1984, in Philadelphia, Pennsylvania"—T.p. verso.
Includes bibliographies and index.
1. Urinary tract infections—Congresses. I. Bondi, Amedeo, 1912- . II. American Society for Microbiology. Eastern Pennsylvania Branch. III. Title. IV. Series. [DNLM: 1. Diagnosis, Laboratory—methods—congresses. 2. Urinary Tract Infections—diagnosis—congresses. 3. Urinary Tract Infections—therapy—congresses. W1 AD559 v.224 / WJ 151 E13u 1984]
RC901.8.E17 1984 616.6 87-35821
ISBN 978-1-4684-8934-7 ISBN 978-1-4684-8932-3 (eBook)
DOI 10.1007/978-1-4684-8932-3

Based on the proceedings of the Eastern Pennsylvania Branch of the American Society for Microbiology Symposium on Urogenital Infections: New Developments in Laboratory Diagnosis and Treatment, held November 15-16, 1984, in Philadelphia, Pennsylvania


Softcover reprint of the hardcover 1st edition 1987
A Division of Plenum Publishing Corporation
233 Spring Street, New York, N.Y. 10013

## ORGANIZING COMMITTEE

### Program Chairman

Amedeo Bondi, Ph.D.
Hahnemann University

### Program Co-Chairman

Joseph M. Campos, Ph.D.
Children's Hospital - National Medical Center

Donald D. Stieritz, Ph.D.
Hahnemann University

### Committee Members

Paul Actor, Ph.D.
Smith Kline & French Laboratories

Josephine Bartola, J.D.
Pennsylvania Department of Health

Walter Ceglowski, Ph.D.
Temple University School of Medicine

Kenneth R. Cundy, Ph.D.
Temple University School of Medicine

Toby K. Eisenstein, Ph.D.
Temple University School of Medicine

Alan T. Evangelista, Ph.D.
Cooper Hospital/University Medical Center

Eileen T. Hinks, Ph.D.
Rolling Hill Hospital

Donald Jungkind, Ph.D.
Thomas Jefferson University

Linda Ann Miller, Ph.D.
Holy Redeemer Hospital and Medical Center

Barbara Zajac, M.D., Ph.D.
Merck Sharp & Dohme

## PREFACE

The purpose of this annual symposium of the Eastern Pennsylvania Branch of the American Society for Microbiology was to organize a panel of scientists to review the many newer aspects of urogenital infections (UGI). From the onset it was recognized that the subject of UGI is a broad one and that it would not be possible to do justice to all aspects in a two day program. Therefore, it was agreed not to attempt an extensive review of the many recognized sexually transmitted diseases (STD), in that these have been the subject of other recent scientific symposia either individually or collectively.

The major goal of this meeting was to review the many newer aspects of UGI relating to the pathogenesis of infections, newer treatment modalities, and newer approaches to the laboratory diagnosis of the respective diseases. The sessions were organized primarily along the lines of different etiologic agents of UGI.

The opening session presented an overview of UGI, with major emphasis on new therapeutic modalities. This area has expanded greatly in recent years because of a better understanding of the etiology of such infections as well as the availability of newer effective chemotherapeutic agents.

The second session presented newer approaches to pathogenesis and treatment with emphasis on experimental animal studies and newer molecular strategies. Subsequent sessions focused on specific causative agents where newer insights have been recently gained. Included were *Chlamydia trachomatis*, *Mycoplasma species*, *Neisseria gonorrhoea* and the ostenisible agent of bacterial vaginosis. The final session focused in a general way on newer approaches to the laboratory diagnosis of the agents of UGI as well as other infections.

All in all the symposium served to review and focus attention on these several newer aspects of UGI with an intended breadth of appeal to the clinician, the basic medical scientist and the clinical microbiologist.

Amedeo Bondi,
Donald D. Stieritz,
Joseph M. Campos and
Linda Ann Miller

ACKNOWLEDGEMENTS

The editors are grateful to the Eastern Pennsylvania Branch of the American Society for Microbiology for sponsoring this symposium and for making this publication possible. The members of the Symposium Committee are also thanked for their diligent work in organizing a successful symposium.

We would like to acknowledge the support and sponsorship of the Bureau of Laboratories of the Pennsylvania Department of Health, Temple University School of Medicine, Hahnemann University, The Medical College of Pennsylvania, the University of Pennsylvania and Thomas Jefferson University.

This symposium would not have been possible without the financial support of the following companies: Abbott Laboratories, Burroughs-Wellcome & Co., Dupont Diagnostic Systems, Glaxo Inc., Hoechst-Roussel Pharmaceuticals, Inc., Marion Laboratories, Medical Products Division/3M, Pharmacia Diagnostocs. Pfizer, Inc., and Smith Kline Diagnostics. We gratefully acknowledge their contributions.

Special thanks are offered to the Pennsylvania Department of Health-Bureau of Laboratories for generously providing help with mailing and registrations; and to Ms. Maritza Santiago for her assistance in layout and typing of the camera-ready copy of the manuscripts.

CONTENTS

## GONORRHEA AND VAGINITIS



## RELATED TOPICS

## URINARY TRACT INFECTION

P. Weiner and D. Kaye

Department of Medicine
The Medical College of Pennsylvania
Philadelphia, Pennsylvania 19129

### DEFINITIONS

Urinary tract infection exists when bacteria are present in urine in the bladder. Significant bacteriuria ( $\geq 10^5$ organisms/ml of urine) defines the numbers of bacteria in midstream clean voided urine that exceed the numbers usually caused by contamination from the anterior urethra. Urinary tract infections can be categorized anatomically into lower tract infection (i.e. involving the bladder) and upper tract infection (infection in the kidney). Cystitis refers to lower tract infection associated with symptoms of frequency, urgency and/or dysuria. One third of patients with cystitis have asymptomatic upper tract infection. The urethral syndrome refers to symptoms of dysuria, frequency, and/or urgency associated with $<10^5$ bacteria per ml of urine. One third of patients with this syndrome have lower tract bacterial infection with bacteria in the bladder as demonstrated by suprapubic bladder aspiration. Acute pyelonephritis refers to upper tract infection associated with symptoms of fever and flank pain. Symptoms of lower tract infection frequently accompany pyelonephritis. Most urinary tract infection is asymptomatic, i.e. asymptomatic bacteriuria. One third of patients with asymptomatic bacteriuria have upper tract infection.

### EPIDEMIOLOGY

The prevalence of bacteriuria in the neonate is about 1%. It is much more common in boys than girls (1) and is often associated with bacteremia. After infancy and into adult life, the prevalence of bacteriuria in men remains much less than 1%. However, after age 65 the prevalence increases and reaches 5-10% by age 80 (2,3). This increase is attributed at least in part to development of prostatic hypertrophy with obstruction of the bladder outlet.

After infancy, the prevalence of bacteriuria in women increases with increasing age. In school age girls it is about 1%, and in young adult women it is 1-3% (4,5) with at least 10-20% of females experiencing a symptomatic infection at some time during their life. In elderly women the prevalence of infection is about 20% (2,3,5,6). In females, spontaneous cure of infection with spontaneous acquisition of new infection is common. In males, spontaneous acquisition of infection is uncommon; when it occurs, the infection can often be related to urethral catheterization.

## INFECTING ORGANISMS

E. coli is by far the most common pathogen in urinary tract infection in patients without structural abnormalities of the urinary tract (7). The relative frequency of other gram negative bacilli ( Klebsiella, Enterobacter, Proteus, and Pseudomonas), as well as enterococci and staphylococci, increases in patients with abnormalities such as mechanical obstruction, neurogenic bladder, and congenital anomalies. The frequency of these organisms is also increased in patients who develop infection following urologic manipulation. These organisms are also more frequently seen in hospitalized patients, especially with in dwelling catheters (8). Staphylococcus aureus in the urinary tract is often associated with pyleonephritis with intrarenal or perinephric abscess formation and occurs as a complication of bacteremia or endocarditis (9). S. saprophyticus tends to cause infection in young, sexually active women via the ascending route (10). Fungi, especially Candida, tend to colonize the lower tract of patients with in dwelling catheters who are receiving antibiotic therapy. Adenoviruses, especially type 11, have been implicated in hemorrhagic cystitis in children, especially in boys (11,12).

Because only a few serogroups of E. coli cause a high proportion of infections (13), it has been postulated that certain virulence factors associated with these serogroups enhance their capacity to colonize the urinary tract and cause infection (14). Some of the virulence factors are increased adherence to uroepithelial cells (14), resistance to serum bactericidal activity (15), higher quantity of K antigen (13) and hemolysin production (16). Of these, adherence seems to be the most significant (14,17-20). Specifically, fimbriae on E. coli bind to uroepithelial cell receptors. Currently, it is thought that fimbriae attaching to mannosides are important in colonization of the lower tract. These are called MS fimbriae for mannose-sensitive fimbriae, because binding is inhibited in the presence of mannose. P fimbriae, which bind to glycolipid receptors appear to be associated with organisms that cause upper tract infection (21). These are called MR fimbriae for mannose-resistant fimbriae, because binding is not inhibited by mannose.

## PATHOPHYSIOLOGY

There are three possible routes by which bacteria can invade the urinary tract: the ascending, hematogenous and lymphatic routes. The ascending pathway (by way of the urethra) is unquestionably the most common. In women, it has been demonstrated that organisms that cause urinary tract infection colonize the vaginal introitus and peri-urethral area before infection occurs (22). Furthermore, several studies indicate a relationship between sexual intercourse and development of urinary tract infection, presumably because bacteria are forced into the bladder from the above mentioned sites of colonization (23-25). The ascending pathway is clearly the route when infection follows instrumentation of the urethra. For example, a single catheterization causes infection in 1% of ambulatory patients. Furthermore, in patients with indwelling catheters with open drainage, virtually all develop infection within 4 days (26).

Pyelonephritis may occasionally follow hematogenous spread. When this occurs it is probably most often seen with S. aureus bacteremia. There is little clinical evidence to support a significant role of lymphatics as a route in the pathogenesis of urinary tract infection.

Host factors are important in the pathophysiology of urinary tract infection. Although the urethral mucosa is colonized, the bladder is normally sterile. Urine itself may be a defense against infection. Urine will not support growth of many fastidious organisms and under certain conditions may even inhibit growth of uropathogens. Some of these conditions are: high urea levels, low pH, and extremes of osmolality (27). In addition, urine has properties that inhibit white cell chemotaxis and killing ability. The flushing mechanism of the bladder is also protective in clearing bacteria, and there may be additional defenses (28). Local defense mechanisms in the perineal and vaginal areas may also play a role in preventing colonization by uropathogens. It has been suggested by some studies that defective local mechanisms may explain recurrent lower tract infections in some women (29). However, other studies have failed to show enhanced bacterial adherence to vaginal epithelial cells (30) or defective local antibody production in such patients (31). Production of local urinary antibody (IgA and IgG) and systemic antibody (IgM and IgG) aimed at bacterial cell wall antigen, accompanies pyelonephritis. Although such antibody responses can protect against ascending or hematogenous pyelonephritis in experimental animals (32-34), the protective role of this humoral response in man is as yet unclear. Lastly, structural lesions that inhibit the normal flow of urine cause stasis of urine and predispose patients to infection.

## DIAGNOSIS OF URINARY TRACT INFECTION

Clinical symptoms and signs are not reliable in diagnosis of urinary tract infection. Significant bacteriuria commonly occurs in the absence of symptoms (i.e. asymptomatic bacteriuria). Furthermore, among women presenting with symptoms of dysuria, only about two-thirds have significant bacteriuria.

Laboratory diagnosis begins with microscopic examination of the urine. A clean catch midstream urine specimen is centrifuged for 5 minutes at 2000 rpm and the sediment is examined under high power. Ten to 50 white cells per $mm^3$ is considered the upper limit of normal. Since each white cell seen per field represents 5-10 leukocytes/$mm^3$, 5-10 white cells per field represents the upper limit of normal. Higher numbers are suggestive but by no means diagnostic of infection. Pyuria may occur in the absence of infection, and asymptomatic infection may occur in the absence of pyuria. However, pyuria is almost always present with symptomatic infection. The presence of at least one bacterium per oil immersion field on a Gram stained specimen of an uncentrifuged clean catch specimen correlates with $\geq 10^5$ bacteria/ml urine, i.e. significant bacteriuria.

A specimen for culture may be obtained either by midstream clean catch, catheterization of the bladder via the urethra, or suprapubic aspiration. The urethra and periurethral areas are normally colonized with bacteria and are difficult to sterilize before obtaining a voided or catheterized specimen; consequently, the numbers of bacteria are quantitated in an attempt to distinguish infection from contamination. Patients with infection usually have $\geq 10^5$ bacteria/ml in bladder and voided urine. In noninfected patients, the bladder is sterile and voided urine usually contains $< 10^4$ organisms/ml.

In symptomatic patients, a single culture with $\geq 10^5$ organisms/ml indicates a 95% chance of true bacteriuria. Women (and probably men)

**with acute symptoms of lower tract infection and counts $<10^5$ organisms/ml may also have true bacterial infection as documented by suprapubic bladder aspiration (see urethral syndrome).**

**If there are $\geq 10^5$ bacteria/ml in a clean catch urine from an asymptomatic patient, there is an 80% chance that this represents true bacteriuria. If 2 specimens demonstrate $\geq 10^5$ bacteria/ml, the probability increases to 95%. However, if an initial specimen shows $<10^5$ organisms/ml, the probability is high against bacteriuria. For example, 95% of cultures from asymptomatic women with counts between $10^4$-$10^5$/ml represent contamination.**

**Samples obtained by catherization are less likely to be contaminated. A single specimen with $\geq 10^5$ organisms/ml from an asymptomatic patient represents infection 95% of the time. Counts between $10^4$-$10^5$ organisms/ml in catheterized urine from asymptomatic patients indicate significant bacteriuria about 50% of the time. These findings apply only to the Enterobacteriaceae. Gram positive organisms, fungi and bacteria with fastidious growth requirements are often present in the $10^4$-$10^5$/ml range in patients with infection (35).**

## THE URETHRAL SYNDROME

**Among sexually active young women with acute onset of symptoms of dysuria, about 50% have significant bacteriuria with $\geq 10^5$ organisms/ml urine. The remaining 50% have $<10^5$ organisms/ml and the term urethral syndrome has been applied to this group (36). Approximately one third of this group, or 17% of the total group with dysuria, have bacteria in the bladder demonstrated by suprapubic aspirates. These women are considered to have a lower urinary tract infection. Of the remaining patients with the urethral syndrome, some have sterile pyuria, due chiefly to Chlamydia trachomatis urethritis and to a lesser extent N. gonorrhoeae infection, some have vaginitis or herpes infection, and in some (usually without pyuria), the cause is unclear, although Ureaplasma urealyticum is a candidate organism.**

## BACTERIAL PROSTATITIS

Bacterial prostatitis occurs as either an acute or chronic process. The syndromes are distinct in that acute prostatitis does not usually result in chronic prostatitis and chronic prostatitis is not usually preceded by a history of acute prostatitis.

Acute bacterial prostatitis is associated with severe inflammation of the prostate gland. It is characterized by high fever, chills and perineal and back pain. In addition, it is associated with symptoms of dysuria, frequency and/or urgency when the bladder and urethra are secondarily involved (37). Patients may also develop bladder outlet obstruction and urinary retention due to the swelling caused by the inflammatory response. The prostatic fluid contains may leukocytes and the causative organism may be seen on Gram stain and can usually be cultured from urine. Massage of the prostate to obtain secretions is not advised, because this can produce severe pain and precipitate bacteremia. Many antibiotics used for urinary tract infections penetrate adequately into the acutely inflammed prostate. These should be administered in doses that achieve therapeutic blood levels.

Chronic bacterial prostatitis is usually caused by E. coli but other gram negative bacilli, staphylococcal species, and diphtheroids have been frequent isolates in some series (37,38). Many men are asymptomatic. Some patients have perineal discomfort or low back pain. The major clinical manifestations are recurrences of urinary tract infection always caused by the same organism. Rectal examination is frequently unremarkable. Because bacteria in the urethra can contaminate prostatic secretions, diagnosis is made by quantitative cultures of urethral urine ($UB_1$), midstream urine ($UB_2$), prostatic secretions expressed by massage or ejaculation, and urine voided after massage ($UB_3$), at a time that urinary tract infection is not present (39). Methods of quantitation must be used that will detect small numbers of bacteria. If chronic bacterial prostatitis is present, the numbers of bacteria in the prostatic fluid will exceed the numbers in $UB_1$ or $UB_2$ by $\geq 10$ fold. If no prostatic fluid can be obtained, the number of bacteria in the $UB_3$ specimen should be $\geq 10$ fold higher than in the $UB_1$ or $UB_2$ specimens. Chronic bacterial prostatis is difficult to cure since few antibiotics penetrate well into the prostate that is not acutely inflammed. Therefore, this condition is likely to cause relapsing urinary tract infection but there may be long periods of time between relapses. Studies using trimethoprim-sulfamethoxazole, oral carbenicillin or rifampin in combination with trimethoprim for 1-3 months or more have reported variable cure rates of 33% to most patients (40-42). If such therapy fails, alternative therapy consists of managing acute exacerbations or urinary tract infection or using chronic suppressive therapy with one half the normal daily dose of the particular agent. Lastly, transurethral prostatectomy to remove the infected tissue is said to be curative in about 1/3 of cases. Prostatectomy is indicated only if there is evidence of obstruction and the procedure is warranted for the obstruction _per se_.

## INFECTIONS IN CHILDREN

Symptoms of urinary tract infections in young children (i.e. less than 2 years old) are non-specific and are chiefly fever, vomiting and failure to thrive. Vesicoureteral reflux occurs in 30 to 50% of children four or less years of age with urinary tract infection and is less common in older children (1,43). The reflux is caused or exacerbated by the inflammation of the immature vesicoureteral junction produced by the infection. Reflux alone can lead to renal scarring but infection probably increases the damage. Children under four years of age are at the highest risk of scarring and some go on to develop hypertension and end stage renal disease. After the age of four, reflux becomes less common even though infection is present. In the absence of obstruction or reflux, urinary tract infection does not usually have serious sequellae.

## INFECTIONS DURING PREGNANCY

During pregnancy, physiologic changes beginning in the first trimester include dilatation of the ureters and renal pelvis, decreased ureteral peristalsis and decreased bladder tone (44). This probably increases susceptibility to infection and the prevalence of asymptomatic bacteriuria in pregnancy is 4-7% (45,46). About 75% of women who develop bacteriuria during pregnancy, have it during the first trimester. About 20% of patients with bacteriuria during pregnancy develop acute pyelonephritis later in the pregnancy (47,48).

Acute pyelonephritis often results in premature delivery. Asymptomatic bacteriuria may also, but less commonly, result in premature delivery. Since the association of asymptomatic bacteriuria with subsequent pyelonephritis is well-established, and since most bacteriuria of pregnancy occurs early in the pregnancy, screening for bacteriuria in the first trimester of pregnancy is advisable with treatment of infected women.

## NATURAL HISTORY OF URINARY TRACT INFECTION IN NON-PREGNANT ADULTS

There is no evidence to suggest that infection in adults, in the absence of other urinary tract abnormalities (most notably obstruction), leads to significant renal disease. Consequently, the major goal of therapy is the elimination of symptoms.

## THERAPY

In choosing antimicrobial therapy, there is no evidence to support use of bactericidal drugs over bacteriostatic agents. Sterilization of the urine requires levels of antibiotic in the urine above the minimal inhibitory concentration for the organism. Such urine levels are achieved after oral administration of virtually all agents commonly used for urinary tract infection. In general, it is not necessary to achieve inhibitory blood levels of the antimicrobial agent. The exception is in treating pyelonephritis with associated bacteremia. One of the most important criteria in selecting an agent is to choose the least toxic, effective drug available.

There are four possible responses to therapy: cure, persistence, relapse, and reinfection. Cure is defined as a negative urine culture on therapy and at follow-up at 1-2 weeks. Persistence refers to significant bacteriuria after 24-48 hours of therapy and means that the urine level of the antibiotic is too low (i.e. not inhibitory). Relapse means response but that the same bacteria returns in significant titers within 1-2 weeks of stopping therapy and usually indicates that the organism has persisted in the urinary tract. Relapse is associated with renal infection, a prostatic nidus of infection (i.e. chronic bacterial prostatitis), and structural abnormalities of the urinary tract (e.g. calculi or obstruction). Apparent relapses are sometimes actually due to a new infection (reinfection) with the same organism. Delayed relapses (greater than 1-2 weeks after initial therapy) are likely to be due to reinfection or to infection of the bladder from chronic bacterial prostatitis. Reinfection is a new infection from outside the urinary tract (i.e. from the urethra).

## ACUTE PYELONEPHRITIS

Patients with symptoms of upper tract infection, who are severely ill should be hospitalized to receive parenteral therapy for possible bacteremia. In addition to a culture, a Gram stain of the urine should be obtained. If gram negative bacilli are seen on Gram stain, our preference is for a combination of a cephalosporin (eg, cefazolin, 1-2g IV every 8 hours) and an aminoglycoside (e.g., gentamicin, 1.7 mg/kg every 8 hours) IV or IM. An alternative is the use of a "third generation" cephalosporin (e.g., cefotaxime 2g IV every 4-6 hours or ceftizoxime 2 g IV every 6-8 hours), which avoids the nephrotoxicity and ototoxicity of the aminoglycoside. When the susceptibility pattern of the organism is known, therapy can be modified to the least expensive, least toxic, single agent available. Once a clinical response occurs, therapy can be completed with an oral agent. In less ill patients, an oral agent (e.g.amoxicillin, cephalexin or trimethoprim-sulfamethoxazole) can be used from the outset. Lack of response of fever or persistently positive blood cultures past the third day of therapy suggests urinary obstruction, intrarenal abscess or perinephric abscess; evaluation of these possibilities requires a renal ultrasound, an intravenous pyelogram and/or an abdominal CT scan. All men and children should be evaluated by ultrasound and perhaps intravenous pyelography to exclude anatomic abnormalities.

Therapy should be continued for 14 days for upper tract infection. Follow-up cultures are recommended at 1-2 weeks to evaluate for relapse.

SYMPTOMATIC LOWER TRACT INFECTION

In women with frequency, urgency and/or dysuria and $\geq 10^5$ bacteria/ml urine, a short course of antimicrobial therapy has been highly effective. In fact, high cure rates have been obtained with single doses of amoxicillin, 3 g orally (49,50), trimethoprim-sulfamethoxazole, one double strength tablet orally (51), and cefonicid, 1g intramuscularly (52). It is likely that virtually any appropriate agent used in treatment of lower urinary tract infection would be effective if given for 24-48 hours. Short course or single dose therapy should be limited to women with less than 7 days of symptoms prior to therapy (53) and should not be used in patients with structural abnormalities, diabetes, or in complicated infection. Such therapy has not yet been adequately evaluated in men or children. Lower tract infections in men and children should probably be treated with 7-10 day conventional courses of antimicrobial therapy. In a sexually active woman with dysuria, who has pyuria but $< 10^5$ bacteria/ml urine, the most likely diagnosis is urinary tract infection or <u>Chlamydia</u> urethritis.

Therefore, if pyuria and bacteriuria are present on a stain of a midstream clean catch urine specimen, a female should receive single dose or short course therapy (e.g. one double strength trimethoprim-sulfamethoxazole tablet, 3g of amoxicillin in a single dose or amoxicillin or cephalexin given in usual dosage for 1-2 days). If pyuria is present but bacteria are not seen on smear (i.e. $<10^5$ organisms/ml), herpes genitalis and vaginitis should first be excluded. Single dose or short course therapy is then a reasonable first approach. If there is no clinical response and subsequently the culture shows $< 10^5$ bacteria/ml, tetracycline, 500mg orally four times a day, should be given for one week to empirically treat for <u>Chlamydia</u> urethritis and gonorrhea. (Cultures or stains for <u>Chlamydia</u> would be ideal but are expensive). If no clinical response occurs and culture shows $\geq 10^5$ organisms/ml, the organism is probably resistant and therapy with a different agent should be tried. Follow-up culture in 1-2 weeks is recommended to detect relapses. Initial response followed by a symptomatic relapse should be treated for 2 weeks for presumptive upper tract infection, but treatment of an asymptomatic relapse is not mandatory in a non-pregnant adult.

ASYMPTOMATIC BACTERIURIA

In general, therapy for asymptomatic bacteriuria is reserved for children and pregnant adults. In contrast, non-pregnant adults usually do not require therapy.

RELAPSING INFECTION

Relapses after therapy are usually due to renal infection, a structural abnormality or chronic bacterial prostatitis. Patients who relapse after single dose or short course therapy for lower tract infection should be retreated for 14 days with the assumption that upper tract infection is present. Further symptomatic relapses or asymptomatic relapses in children or pregnant women should be pursued with studies to exclude surgically correctable lesions. Adults who relapse with symptoms or pregnant women or children who relapse without symptoms after 2 weeks of treatment, should be considered for 6 weeks or even longer therapy (54).

REINFECTION

Infrequent reinfections with lower tract symptoms should be treated with individual single-dose or short courses of therapy. Patients with frequent symptomatic reinfections should be considered for long term prophylaxis. In addition, frequent asymptomatic reinfections in children or pregnant females should be considered for long term prophylaxis. Trimethoprim-sulfamethoxazole, trimethoprim alone and nitrofurantoin are useful agents for prophylaxis because emergence of resistant bacteria is unlikely even with prolonged use (55-57). Doses are usually given once a day in the evening and are low (e.g. one half of a trimethoprim-sulfamethoxazole tablet or 50 mg nitrofurantoin). Single-dose prophylaxis (with similar low doses) before sexual intercourse can decrease the number of reinfections in women who develop frequent reinfections in association with intercourse (58).

REFERENCES


1. F.G. Boineau, J.E. Lewy. Urinary tract infection in children: An overview. Pediatr. Ann. 64: 515 (1975).
2. D. Kaye. Urinary tract infection in the elderly. Bull. NY. Acad. Med. 56: 209, (1980).
3. J.M. Romano, D. Kaye. UTI in the elderly: Common yet atypical. Geriatrics 36:113 (1981).
4. L.R. Freedman, J.P. Phair, M. Seki, H.B. Hamilton, M.D. Nefzger and M. Hirata. The epidemiology of urinary tract infections in Hiroshima. Yale J. Biol. Med. 37: 262 (1965).
5. E.H. Kass, W. Savage, B.A.G. Santamarina. The significance of bacteriuria in preventive medicine, in E.H. Kass (ed): Progress in Pyelonephritis. Philadelphia, F.A., Davis, p. 3. (1965).
6. J.P. Sanford. Urinary tract symptoms and infection. Ann. Rev. Med. 26: 485 (1975).
7. J.C. Gould. The comparative bacteriology of acute and chronic urinary tract infection, in O'Grady, F., Brumfitt, W. (eds): Urinary Tract Infection, London, Oxford Univ. Press, p. 43. (1968).
8. M. Turck, W.E. Stamm. Nosocomial infection of the urinary tract. Am. J. Med. 70: 651 (1981).
9. L.E. Cluff, R.C. Reynolds, D.L. Page and J.L. Breckenridge. Staphylococcal bacteremia and altered host resistance. Ann. Intern. Med. 69: 859 (1968).
10. P.A. Jordon, A. Iravani, G.A. Richard and H. Baer. Urinary tract infection caused by Staphylococcus saprophyticus. J. Infect. Dis. 142: 510 (1980).
11. M.A. Mufson, L.M. Zollar, V.N. Mandad and D. Manalo. Adenovirus infection in acute hemorrhagic cystitis: A study in 25 children. Am. J. Dis. Child. 121: 281 (1971).
12. Y.N. Namazaki, T. Kumasaka, N. Yana, M. Yamanaka, T. Miyazawa, S. Takai and N. Ishida. Further study on acute hemorrhagic cystitis due to adenovirus. N. Eng. J. Med. 289: 344 (1973).
13. A.P. Roberts and R. Phillips. Bacteria causing symptomatic urinary tract infection or bacteriuria. J. Clin. Pathol. 32: 492 (1979).
14. C. Svanborg-Eden, L. Hagberg, L.A. Hanson, T. Korhonen, H. Leffler and S. Olling. Adhesion of Escherichia coli in urinary tract infection. CIBA Found. Symp., 80: 161 (1981).

15. B. Bjorksten, and B. Kaijser. Interaction of human serum and neutrophils with Escherichia coli strains: Differences between strains isolated from urine of patients with pyelonephritis or asymptomatic bacteriuria. Infect. Immun. 22: 308 (1978).
16. C. Hughes, J. Hacker, A. Roberts and W. Goebel. Hemolysin production as a virulence marker in symptomatic and asymptomatic urinary tract infections caused by Escherichia coli. Infect. Immun. 39: 546 (1983).
17. C. Svanborg-Eden, E.C. Gotschlich, T.K. Korhonen, H. Leffler and G. Schoolnik. Aspects of structure and function of pili of uropathogenic E. coli. Prog. Allergy 33: 189 (1983).
18. L. Hagberg, R. Hull, S. Hull, S. Falkow, R. Freter and C. Svanborg Eden. Contribution of adhesin to bacterial persistence in the mouse urinary tract. Infect. Immun. 40: 265 (1983).
19. L. Hagberg, U. Jodal, T.K. Korhonen. G. Lidin-Janson, U. Lindberg and C. Svanborg Eden. Adhesion, haemagglutination and virulence of Escherichia coli causing urinary tract infections. Infect. Immun. 31: 564 (1981).
20. C. Svanborg-Eden, B. Eriksson, and L.A. Hanson. Adhesion of Escherichia coli to human uroepithelial cells in vitro. Infect. Immun. 18: 767 (1977).
21. H. Lefler, and C. Svanborg-Eden. Glycolipid receptors for uropathogenic Escherichia coli binding to human erythrocytes and uroepithelial cells. Infect. Immun. 34: 930 (1981).
22. T.A. Stamey, M. Timothy, M. Millar, et al. Recurrent urinary tract infections in adult women. The role of introital enterobacteria. Calif. Med. 115: 1 (1976).
23. R.M. Buckley, M. McGuckin, and R.R. MacGregor. Urine bacterial counts following sexual intercourse. N. Engl. J. Med. 298: 321 (1978).
24. M.C. Kelsey, M.G. Mead, R.N. Gruneberg and J.D. Oriel. Relationship between sexual intercourse and urinary tract infection in women attending a clinic for sexually transmitted diseases. J. Med. Microbiol. 12: 511 (1979).
25. L.E. Nicolle, G.K.M. Harding, J. Preiksaitis and A.R. Ronald. The association of urinary tract infection with sexual intercourse. J. Infect. Dis. 146: 579 (1982).
26. E.H. Kass. Asymptomatic infections of the urinary tract. Trans. Assoc. Am. Physicians. 69: 56 (1956).
27. D. Kaye. Antibacterial activity of human urine. J. Clin. Invest. 47: 2374 (1968).
28. C.E. Cox and F. Hinman, Jr. Experiments with induced bacteriuria, vesical emptying and bacterial growth on the mechanism of bladder defense to infection. J. Urol. 86: 739 (1961).
29. T.A. Stamey. The role of introital enterobacteria in recurrent urinary infections. J. Urol. 109: 467 (1973).
30. C.L. Parsons and J.D. Schmidt. In vitro bacterial adherence to vaginal cells of normal and cystitis prone women. J. Urol. 123: 184 (1980).
31. L.M. Kurdydyk, K. Kelley, G.K.M. Harding, P. Mirwaldt, L. Thompson, F.J. Buckwold and A.R. Ronald. The role of cervico-vaginal antibody in the pathogenesis of recurrent urinary tract infection in women. Infect. Immun. 29: 76 (1980).
32. B. Kaijser, P. Larson, S. Olling and R. Schneerson. Protection against acute pyelonephritis caused by Escherichia coli in rats, using isolated capsular antigen conjugated to bovine serum albumin. Infect. Immun. 39: 142 (1983).
33. L.A. Hanson, A. Fasth, U. Jodal, B. Kaijser and C. Svanborg Eden. Biology and pathology of urinary tract infection. J. Clin. Pathol. 34: 695 (1981).

34. I. Mattsby-Balfzer, L.A. Hanson, S. Olling and B. Kaijser. Experimental Escherichia coli ascending infection in rats: Active peroral immunization with live Escherichia coli. Infect. Immun. 35: 647 (1982).
35. V.T. Andriole. Diagnosis of urinary tract infections by culture, In Kaye D (ed): Urinary Tract Infection and its Management. St. Louis, CV Mosby, 28 (1972).
36. D.J. Gallager, J.Z. Montgomerie, and J.D. North. Acute infections of the urinary tract and the urethral syndrome in general practice. Br. Med. J. 5413: 622 (1965).
37. E.M. Meares: Prostatitis: A review. Urol. Clin. North Am. 2: 3, (1975).
38. G.W. Drach. Prostatitis: Man's hidden infection. Urol. Clin. North Am. 3: 499 (1975).
39. E.M. Meares and T.A. Stamey. Bacteriological localization patterns in bacterial prostatitis and urethritis. Invest. Urol. 5: 492 (1968).
40. E.M. Meares. Long-term therapy of chronic bacterial prostatitis with trimethoprim-sulfamethoxazole. Can. Med. Assoc. J. 112: 225 (1975).
41. D.F. Mobley. Bacterial prostatitis: Treatment with carbenicillin indanyl sodium. Invest. Urol. 19: 31 (1981).
42. H. Giamarellou, J. Kosmidis, M. Leonidas, M. Papadakis and G.K. Daikos. A study of the effectiveness of rifampin in chronic prostatitis caused mainly by Staphylococcus aureus. J. Urol. 128: 321 (1982).
43. J. Smellie, D. Edwards, N. Hunter, I.C.S. Normand and N. Prescod. Vesico-ureteral reflux and renal scarring. Kidney Int. 8: 565 (1975).
44. V.T. Andriole. Urinary tract infection in pregnancy. Urol. Clin. North Am. 2: 485 (1975).
45. C.W. Norden and E.H. Kass. Bacteriuria of pregnancy: A critical appraisal. Ann. Rev. Med. 19: 431 (1968).
46. C.W. Norden. Significance and management of bacteriuria of pregnancy, in D. Kaye (ed): Urinary Tract Infection and its Management. St. Louis, CV Mosby, p. 171, (1972).
47. E. Kass. Bacteriuria and pyelonephritis of pregnancy. Trans. Assoc. Am. Physician 72: 257 (1959).
48. A. Kincaid-Smith and M. Bullen. Bacteriuria in pregnancy. Lancet 1: 395 (1965).
49. L.S.T. Fang, N.E. Tolokoff-Rubin and R.H. Rubin. Efficacy of single-dose and conventional amoxicillin therapy in urinary-tract infection localized by the antibody coated bacteria technic. N. Engl. J. Med. 298: 413 (1978).
50. R.H. Rubin, L.S.T. Fang, S.R. Jones, R.S. Munford, J.M. Slepack, P.A. Varga, L. Onheiber, C.L. Hall and N.E. Tolkoff-Rubin. Single dose amoxicillin therapy for urinary tract infection. J.A.M.A. 244: 561 (1980).
51. R.R. Bailey and G.D. Abbott. Treatment of urinary tract infection with a single dose of trimethoprim-sulfamethoxazole. Can. Med. Assoc. J. 118: 551 (1978).
52. R.E. Pontzer, R.E. Krieger, J.A. Boscia, W. McNamee, M.E. Levison and D. Kaye. Single-dose cefonicid therapy for urinary tract infections. Antimicrob. Agents and Chemother. 23: 814 (1983).
53. W.E. Stamm. Single-dose treatment of cystitis. J.A.M.A. 244: 591 (1980).
54. M. Turck, A.R. Ronald and R.G. Petersdorf. Relapse and reinfection in chronic bacteriuria. II. The correlation between site of infection and pattern of recurrence in chronic bacteriuria. N. Engl. J. Med. 278: 422 (1968).

55. T.A. Stamey, M. Condy and G. Mihara. Prophylactic efficacy of nitrofurantoin macrocrystals and trimethoprim-sulfamethoxazole in urinary infection. N. Engl. J. Med. 296: 780 (1977).
56. R.B. Light, A.R. Ronald, G.K.M. Harding, J. Dikkema, L. Thompson and F.J. Buckwold. Trimethoprim alone in the treatment and prophylaxis of urinary tract infection. Arch. Intern. Med. 141: 1807 (1981).
57. R.N. Gruneberg, J.M. Smellie, A. Leaky and W.S. Atkin. Long-term, low-dose, co-trimoxazole in prophylaxis of childhood urinary tract infection: Bacteriologic aspects. Brit. Med. J. 2: 206 (1976).
58. K. Vosti. Recurrent urinary tract infection: Prevention by prophylactic antibiotics after sexual intercourse. J.A.M.A. 231: 934 (1975).

## CRITICAL ISSUES IN THE DIAGNOSIS OF UROGENITAL INFECTIONS

Richard C. Tilton

Professor of Laboratory Medicine
University of Connecticut Health Center
Farmington, CT 06032

The clinician and the laboratorian are aware of the wide variety of new and innovative methods for the diagnosis of urogenital disease. Subsequent papers in this volume will provide methodologic and analytical precision and accuracy of a variety of instruments and techniques for diagnosis. This review will focus on 3 areas of interest: a) a broad overview of technology, b) the relevance of laboratory data, and c) practical considerations of Beysian statistics as they apply to microbiology.

### TECHNOLOGY ASSESSMENT

The Gram stain may be the best screening method available for urogenital disease. There are a number of reports on the use of the Gram stain and acridine orange stains for screening for significant bacteriuria. However, laboratory acceptance has been slow since the procedure is labor intensive, albeit economical. Cellular components, such as leukocytes, also reflect infection. Additionally, a variety of chemical tests have been proposed over the past 40 or 50 years. The ones currently in vogue are leukocyte esterase and nitrite. These tests are effective in some laboratories and not in others. One can also detect bacteria or cellular components in the spun sediment. Sediment examination for either bacteria or leukocytes is suitable only for crude qualitative results.

There are other more automated methods to detect urinary tract infection. One such instrument, is the Marion Scientific Co. Bactiscreen. It is a very simple instrument in the category of "Why didn't I think of that, because it is so obvious and apparently so lucrative." The Bactiscreen, in 2-3 minutes, filters urine through a filter pad and stains it with safranin. The pink color of the filter pad is roughly proportional to the concentration of bacteria in the urine specimen.

The Abbott MS2 and the General Diagnostics Autobac, which have been used for antimicrobial susceptibility and identification of bacteria can also be used for urine screening. They are relatively sensitive and specific. The instruments however are expensive and the time required for the test is excessive (2-3 hours). If you have an instrument, it may be worth using at a cost of about 12¢ per specimen to screen urine. The Vitek AMS is in the same category, except it does comprehensive bacteriology directly on the urine. How well it performs is open to conjecture. Although there are currently two ATP analyzers for urine screening, ATP analysis has not caught on. Initially, the instruments were unreliable. Subsequently, there was interference from host ATP. Nevertheless, ATP analysis is available for urinary tract infection screening. It is sensitive, specific, and rapid.

There are a number of methods for localization of urinary tract infection including bladder washout, ureteral catheterization, (both invasive), the antibody coated bacteria (ACB) test, C-Reactive Protein (CRP), and specific antibodies to uropathogens. ACB tests are presently in disfavor due to problems of both sensitivity and specificity. CRP is non-specific and some of our studies indicate that specific antibody is not reliable for localization of UTI.

There are a number of tests available for Chlamydia. They include Chlamydiazyme (Abbott), and other enzyme immunoassays. At present, the Chlamydiazyme suffers from lack of sensitivity in male patients. The direct fluorescent antibody (DFA) test from SYVA, and others, is both sensitive and specific although it does not lend itself to batch processing. There will soon be a DNA probe available for chlamydia, and a number of other companies are developing enzyme immunoassays for direct identification of chlamydia.

Fung et al (1) evaluated a DNA probe for HSV 1 (Enzo) and compared it with fluorescent microscopy (Electronucleonics, Inc.), both performed on the direct specimen. When compared with tissue culture, the probe lacked sensitivity (89.5%) and was not totally specific (86.3%). The fluorescent method showed adequate but not outstanding sensitivity (78.9%) and excellent specificity (100%).

Gonozyme (Abbott), the EIA for *Neisseria gonorrhoeae* has been widely tested. Most investigators have reported that it lacked either sensitivity, specificity, or both in females but was highly sensitive and specific for males. Of course, so is the Gram stain of urethral exudate, at least for males. A number of companies are developing EIA methods for the direct detection of *N. gonorrhoeae* in clinical specimens. There are, as well, numerous methods for the rapid identification of the isolate from a primary plate.

The mere availability of a test is not a primary justification for its use. Funding priorities are changing and laboratories are becoming fiscal millstones instead of revenue bonanzas. It is essential, then, for both the laboratory and the clinician to examine the relevance of the data that is generated. Two clinical syndromes, bacterial vaginosis and acute cystitis, can be used to demonstrate the point. On the one hand, to cite examples when laboratory tests may not be relevant, and on the other hand, to provide instances when laboratory testing may not be economical and perhaps should not be used.

Bacterial vaginosis was formerly called non-specific vaginitis and was thought to be caused solely by *Gardnerella*. Bacterial vaginosis is not caused by *Gardnerella*, but by *Gardnerella* and an anaerobic Gram negative rod called *Mobiluncus*. Eschenbach (2), in a provocative paper, indicated that clinical diagnosis was preferred. That is, homogeneous appearance of the exudate, a pH of the exudate greater than 4.5 and a fishy or amine-like odor when KOH is added to the specimen. Clue cells are also important diagnostic indicators. A Gram stain in a patient with bacterial vaginosis reveals a prevalence of Gram variable rods suggestive of Gardnerella. The normal vaginal flora changes in bacterial vaginosis. Culture of G. vaginalis is not a reliable predictor of disease.

Eschenbach (2) states that "Bacterial vaginitis can be diagnosed using a variety of criteria. Except for research, the diagnosis should not involve the use of culture for either Gardnerella or for anaerobic organisms. Gardnerella can be recovered from 40% of women without vaginal infection and from 40% of women after successful therapy for bacterial vaginosis. Thus, culture is both non-sensitive and non-specific. Reliance on the presence or absence of Gardnerella has led to major misconceptions in the diagnosis and treatment of this condition. The continued use of diagnostic criteria based solely upon whether Gardnerella is present or absent leads to unnecessary concern and treatment of a large number of women who are simply colonized with Gardnerella. Similarly, anaerobic cultures are too nonspecific and expensive to be widely used. Therefore, the main thrust of diagnosis is to identify evidence of bacterial vaginosis without using culture methods."

The second example is taken from a paper by Schultz et al. (3). He evaluated single dose versus multiple dose therapy using trimethoprim-sulfamethoxazole therapy on a group of women with acute cystitis. As an adjunct to this trial, the investigator evaluated the role of laboratory testing in the diagnosis of acute cystitis. He indicated that the average direct cost in Minnesota of seeing a patient with acute cystitis was $79.49. The laboratory was responsible for 66% of the cost, the physician, 22%, and medication, 12%.

Patients responded to trimethoprim-sulfamethoxazole regardless of initial bacterial colony counts. In the study, there was no relationship of hematuria and pyuria to treatment outcome. Schultz stated "Pyuria does not reliably predict treatment outcome. There is no correlation between the outcome and the presence or absence of hematuria."

The conclusions were that routine urinalysis and culture were not necessary in selected women who were non-pregnant, 18-55 years old, no pyelonephritis, no diabetes, and no recent urinary tract infections.

The point is that there is controversy as to whether laboratory data is useful, or even desirable, in some circumstances. It would be unfortunate, then, in such an overview, not to mention the predictive value of diagnostic tests. Ferraro and Kuntz (4) state "In general, until recent years, clinical microbiologic tests have not been characterized or evaluated in other than the classical terms of sensitivity and specificity." These characterizations are, by themselves, inadequate for realistic appraisal of the goodness of a diagnostic test. The usefulness of a test depends not only on the sensitivity and specificity but also on the prevalence of the disease in the population and the predictive value. It has not become apparent that an appreciation of the sensitivity and specificity of a particular test may be useless or even misleading without some knowledge of the prevalence of the particular disease in the population for which the diagnostic test is intended.

There are complex relationships between sensitivity, specificity, prevalence, and predictive value. As the specificity of a test decreases, the value of the test is not in a positive result but in a negative one. As the prevalence of disease in the population increases, the goodness of a positive result increases. This is assuming specificity and sensitivity remain the same. The corollary is that as the sensitivity of the test decreases, the true value of a test is in a positive result. This is assuming high specificity. However, as the disease prevalence increases, the goodness of a negative result increases. The predictive value of a test can be improved by one or more of the following: The specificity of a test can be increased by improving the test technology. As the specificity increases, the predictive value positive increases. Another method is to increase the apparent disease prevalence in the patients to be tested by doing one of two things, either preselecion of the population to be tested, or testing of a higher risk group.

REFERENCES


1. J.C. Fung, J. Shanley, and R.C. Tilton. Comparison of the Detection of HSV in Direct Clinical Specimens using HSV-specific DNA Probes and Monoclonal Antibodies. Abstr. Ann. Mtng. Am. Soc. Microbiol. S9, p. 283 (1985).
2. D.A. Eschenbach. Diagnosis of Bacterial Vaginosis: Role of the Laboratory. Clin. Micro. Newsl. 6, 134-138 (1984).
3. H.J. Shultz, McCaffrey, T.F. Keys and F.T. Nobrega. Acute Cystitis: A Prospective Study of Laboratory Tests and Duration of Therapy. Mayo Clin. Proc. 59, 391-397 (1984).
4. M.J.B. Ferraro, and L.J.Kuntz. Predictive Value of the Microbiologic Diagnostic Tests, pp. 248-253, in "Significance of Medical Microbiology in the Care of Patients," 2nd ed. V.J. Lorian. Williams and Wilkins, Baltimore (1982)

# CONTROVERSIES IN URINARY TRACT INFECTION

S. Grant Mulholland and Kenneth Weisman

Department of Urology
Jefferson Medical College
Philadelphia, PA 19107

There has been some controversy in the past concerning the pathogenesis of urinary tract infection. The routes of infection considered to be of significance are: the ascending or retrograde route; the lymphatic route; and the hematogenous route. It is now felt that the urinary tract, especially in the female, is infected in a retrograde fashion. The female is autoinfected from her own stool. The bacteria colonize the perineum then progress to the vagina, urethra, bladder and possibly the kidneys. In an infection prone female, the prelude to the infection is colonization of the vagina with gram negative bacteria (1). In the female who does not have a history of urinary tract infection or who is not prone to urinary tract infection, colonization of the vagina with typical urinary pathogens is not a common event.

The male has a long urethra in which the bacterial count gets progressively less as one goes from the meatus to the bladder neck. Possibly in the male, other routes of infection might become important. The prostatic fluid has been shown to be antibacterial. The female is definitely more prone to urinary tract infection. The female urethra has a short length, approximately 3 to 4 cms. The distal aspect of the urethra is bathed in bacteria and as one goes up the urethra, the counts decrease. There is turbulent flow in the urethra which may reflux bacteria up into the bladder with voiding. Sexual activity milks bacteria back into the bladder. Also, the female with hormonal changes of menstruation and menopause has changes in the lining cells of the urethra. Embryologically, the cells in the urethra are related to the cells in the vagina. With a decrease in estrogen and progesterone, there is atrophy of the lining cells and substances they secrete predisposing to bacterial colonization (2).

The bladder has the ability to remain sterile in a very efficient manner due to the following properties:

1. The washing action of urine flow.
2. Antibacterial properties of the bladder mucosa.
3. Antibacterial properties of the urine.

There is no doubt that the washing action is probably the most important. If the bacteria are not allowed to adhere to the bladder mucosa and therefore cannot remain behind after voiding, they are very efficiently swept out, and the bladder is kept sterile. When there is no obstruction or abnormality to urine flow, it is actually difficult to experimentally maintain an infection in the laboratory animal. It has been shown in our laboratory that the mucopolysaccharide coating of the bladder acts as an antiadherence substance. When this substance is present and normal, the bacteria cannot stick and are swept away quite efficiently (3).

It is curious that the incidence of urinary tract infection in the female rises after menopause and if one plots this incidence of infection against secretion of estrogen and progesterone, they have an inverse relationship. As the estrogen and progesterone secretion decrease, the incidence of urinary tract infection increases. This is presumably due to atrophy of the cells and also a decrease in the mucopolysaccharide coating. It has been shown experimentally that if one oophorectomizes animals, they do not handle urinary tract infection as well as normal female animals (2). Also, it has been shown histologically, that after oophorectomy, the mucopolysaccharide layer decreases quantitatively (4).

There also has been a considerable amount of work done on certain bacterial receptor sites within the bladder for bacterial organisms, especially E. coli (5,6). It has been shown that infection prone women have a preponderance of certain P-antigens on their cell surfaces which may be different from the normal population. This might suggest that the tendency for a female to develop a urinary tract infection may be an inherited problem due to the antigen configuration of her uroepithelial cells.

In order to thoroughly understand all aspects of urinary tract infection, one should be well acquainted with the natural history of this infection in both the male and the female. As far as the male is concerned, there is a very low incidence of urinary tract infection between the newborn age and 40 years of age. The male does have a slight increase in incidence in the neonatal period (7). This is usually associated with prematurity, neonatal sepsis, etc. Usually these infections do not originate within the urinary tract but are metastatic from some other place. At the age of 40, things begin to go wrong with the male, both medically and urologically. All of the diseases which begin to occur increase the incidence of urinary tract infection. Therefore, there is a gradual rise in the incidence of urinary tract infection, beginning around the age of 40-45. All bacterial infections in the male are significant and a great number of these are associated with some type of pathology. Therefore, all bacterial urinary tract infections in the male should be evaluated.

In the female, around the age of one, there is a slight increase in the incidence of urinary tract infection (1-2%). Also at this age, there is high incidence of urinary tract pathology associated with the infection (8,9). A large percentage of this pathology is correctable, therefore, all girls in this age group should be evaluated. As the child enters the elementary school ages, there is a fairly stable incidence of urinary tract infection. These young girls have an infection prevalence of 1% (10). As the child ages, the chance of finding pathology associated with these infections is reduced. It is therefore felt that in the very young child, an evaluation is indicated but as the child gets older, one might not evaluate all of these children, especially if it is a solitary bladder infection. An older child who has two or more infections or evidence of pyelonephritis should be evaluated. There then is a quiescent period in the female as far as urinary tract infection is concerned until puberty. At around the ages of 17 or 18, the incidence increases (3-4%). This incidence is thought to be due to sexual activity, pregnancy, etc. In a study of nuns (11), who presumably are celibate, the incidence is similar to that of school girls. Most infections during this age group do not have to be investigated unless there is: an unusual organism cultured, bleeding, evidence of upper tract infection, resistance to treatment or multiple recurrences. At the age of 50, after menopause, the incidence of infection gradually rises. After the age of 70, approximately one-third of the female population is bacteriuric. This is due to the changes after menopause and also the accumulation of multiple urologic and medical disorders. In this age group, the female should be investigated if there is some suspicion of underlying disease. Usually the high incidence of infection is accepted and evaluation is not aggressive.

Who should be investigated? Essentially all males with a bacterial urinary tract infection should be investigated. Young females with urinary tract infection definitely should be investigated. As the female child gets older the need for investigation is reduced. Older women with urinary tract infection should not be investigated except in specific instances with suspicious signs or symptoms.

This raises another controversy in urinary tract infection; how should a patient be evaluated? Should culture be routinely used in urinary tract infection? If a female has a routine community type of infection, she undoubtedly is autoinfected from her own fecal flora and the infecting organism is E. coli, therefore, the need for culturing in this patient is not necessary. As infections become more recurrent or complicated, different organisms will arise and culturing may be necessary. Also, with exposure to antimicrobials, other species are seen which may be more resistant. Therefore, for the vast majority of infections, the microscope is used to verify the presence of bacteruria, and cultures are not necessary. In the male, cultures may be necessary in almost every infection because of the higher incidence of resistant organisms and different species.

Should an intravenous pyelogram be performed as a routine part of the evaluation (12)? Possibly the best way to obtain information as to the architecture of the upper tracts, presence of pathology, or presence of obstruction is with an intravenous pyelogram or ultrasound. If an intravenous pyelogram is considered more invasive or dangerous, possibly an ultrasound will give enough gross information so that the presence of serious disease can be ruled out.

Cystoscopy has been thought of as part of the evaluation of urinary tract infection but cystoscopy yields a minimal amount of information. In the adult, the information, especially in the adult female, is minimal unless some one has a suspicion of neoplasm or some abnormality in the lower urinary tract. A voiding cystourethrogram in a child is a vital diagnostic study. This demonstrates many abnormalities which may be conducive to urinary tract infection. Isotopes instilled into the bladder can tell us if reflux is present. (One might consider this to be a less invasive study because of less exposure to radiation). Isotopic studies can tell us if there is any gross abnormality or obstruction. The basic evaluation of urinary tract infection now appears to be an intravenous pyelogram, possibly cystoscopy and possibly a cystogram. We are looking for diseases which can be treated, presumably surgically, to reduce the susceptibility to infection.

This raises another controversy in urinary tract infection; how should one treat the infection? The goal of treatment is to sterilize the urine and to relieve the patient of symptoms. It has been shown recently that the time honored methods of treating urinary tract infection are not necessarily correct. In uncomplicated urinary tract infections, especially in the female, a rather short course of treatment, even as short as one pill, can cure an infection (13,14,15,16). If the patient does have some complicating factor, often a longer course is necessary. For more recurrent infections or infections involving the upper tract, longer courses are necessary. Also in patients who have multiple recurrences, prophylactic usage of small doses of antimicrobials may be helpful (17). Success has been seen with utilization of innocuous antimicrobials after intercourse, at bedtime (possibly every other night), and with menstruation. Hydration of the patient, acidification of the urine, etc, all seem to help if one is looking for reduction in recurrent urinary tract infections.

Another controversy is what drug to use. The physician should keep in mind:

1. Cost - There are many antimicrobials which are very inexpensive and can be utilized for the treatment of infection. Often newer drugs are expensive and not necessary. The unnecessary expense of antimicrobials for treatment of urinary tract infection has been estimated in the millions of dollars per year.

2. Availability of the drug - has to be kept in mind although most antimicrobials are readily available to the patient.

3. Tolerance - Ideally the drug should be completely tolerated and have no side effects.

4. Allergy - Allergy is important especially with penicillins and cephalosporins. Other drugs have a low incidence of allergic problems.

5. Untoward reactions - Most of the antimicrobials that we use for urinary tract infection have a few untoward reactions but the physician should be well aware of them.

6. Absorption - Ideally, the antimicrobials that we use for urinary tract infections should be completely absorbed in the upper G.I. tract so that there is no disturbance of the large bowel flora.

7. Serum concentration - Serum concentration of the drug is not important in the treatment of urinary tract infection.

8. Urine concentration - Is extremely important therefore, we should have a drug that is well filtered and/or secreted rapidly in the urinary tract. Almost all of the drugs utilized have very high urine levels.

9. Effects on vaginal and bowel flora - If a drug is well absorbed in the upper G.I. tract, there is little difficulty with disturbance of flora in the vagina and the bowel which would cause diarrhea and vaginitis.

10. The antimicrobial spectrum - Some antimicrobials have a poor gram-negative spectrum and should never be used.

11. Development of resistance - This is quite common with some antimicrobials due to their mechanism of action and/or urine concentration.

12. The mechanism of action - as to whether the drug is cidal or static does not seem to be important in the treatment of urinary tract infection.

If the clinician has a drug which is inexpensive, readily available, well tolerated, associated with no allergic reactions, completely absorbed in the upper G.I. tract, has a rapid high urinary concentration, has no effect on the vaginal or bowel flora, has a good antimicrobial spectrum, and does not have a problem with development of resistance, the clinician has an ideal drug.

In the management of an infection, one should categorize all infections in order to plan treatment; the antimicrobial that should be selected; and also if cultures should be performed. The sex of the patient is extremely important as far as the treatment of infection, whether cultures are necessary and what antimicrobials should be used. The flora in the male and female are certainly different. Whether the infection occurred in the hospital or the community effects the flora and resistance of organisms. An acute infection, especially in the female, is almost undoubtedly an E. coli infection. Recurrent infections often involve more resistant E. coli organisms or different species, because of the exposure to antimicrobials. Chronic infections or infections that never clear are associated with resistant organisms and also multiple species. Infections, that are complicated by either urinary tract disease or medical disease, are often more difficult to treat, not only because of the complicating factor, but also because of the high incidence of more resistant organisms. Whether the urinary tract infection is upper or lower is extremely important as far as selection of the antimicrobial and length of treatment. If one considers all these aspects, the clinician will have a better idea as how to treat the infection.

The last controversy of many that may be present in urinary tract infection is the urethral catheter. As long as a catheter is in place, the urinary tract is contaminated. After introduction of the catheter, there is an incidence of bacteriuria of 4%. As days go by, a greater percentage of patients with an indwelling catheter become infected. The clinician must accept this infection. If the infection endangers the patient's life, it must be treated. An example would be the immunosuppressed patient who is catheterized. This patient is in a hospital environment and will be exposed to resistant organisms. In order to clear bacteriuria while a catheter is in place, one must use very aggressive treatment. Using antimicrobials to "cover" the catheter, is useless and serves no purpose. This is commonly done in hospitals and in outpatients. The bacteria are never eradicated. After removal of the catheter, one may want to treat the patient with a short course of antimicrobials to clear the urine and have the patient symptom-free in a relatively short period of time.

REFERENCES

1. T.A. Stamey. The role of introital enterobacteria in recurrent urinary infections. J. Urol. 109: 467 (1973).
2. S.G. Mulholland, S.K. Qureshi, R.W. Fritz, and H. Silverman. Effect of hormonal deprivation on the bladder defense mechanism. J. Urol. 127: 1010-1013 (1982).
3. C.L. Parsons, C. Greenspan, S.W. Moore, and S.G. Mulholland. Role of surface mucin in primary antibacterial defense of bladder. Urol. 9: 48 (1977).

4. K. Weisman, H. Callahan, H. Cooper, R. Fritz. and S.G. Mulholland. Decrease in rabbit mucosal glycoproteins after oophorectomy. J. Urol. 132: 380-383 (1984).
5. C. Svanborg-Eden and H. Leffler. Glycosphigolipids of human urinary tract epithelial cells as possible receptors for adhering Escherichia coli bacteria. Scand. J. Dis. Suppl. 24: 144 (1980).
6. S.G. Mulholland, M. Mooreville and C.L. Parsons. Urinary tract infections and P blood group antigens. Urol. 24: 232-235 (1984).
7. T.A. Stamey. Urinary infections in infancy and childhood, Chapter 6, pgs. 290-294 in Pathogenesis and Treatment of Urinary Tract Infections, T.A. Stamey, (ed.), Williams & Willaims, Baltimore/London (1980).
8. J. Winberg, H.J. Andersen, T. Bergstrom, B. Jacobsson, H. Larson and K. Lincoln. Epidemiology of symptomatic urinary tract infection in childhood. Acta. Paediatr. Scan. (suppl.) 252: 3 (1974).
9. G.L. Rolleston, F.T. Shannon, and W.L.F. Utley. Relationship of infantile vesicoureteric reflux to renal damage. Br. Med. J. 1: 460 (1970).
10. C.M. Kunin. An overview of urinary tract infection, pgs. 39-47 in Detection, Prevention and Management of Urinary Tract Infections, C.M. Kunin, (ed.), 3rd edition. Lea & Feibinger, Philadelphia, PA (1979).
11. C.M. Kunin, and R.C. McCormack. An epidemiologic study of bacteriuria and blood pressure among nuns and working women. N. Engl. J. Med. 278: 635-642 (1968).
12. W.R. Fair, B.L. McClennan and R.G. Jost. Are excretory urograms necessary in evaluating women with urinary tract infection? J. Urol. 121: 313 (1979).
13. W.R. Fair, D.B. Crane, L.J. Peterson, C. Dahmer, B. Tague, and W. Amos. Three day treatment of urinary tract infections. J. Urol. 123: 717 (1980).
14. D.I. Rosen. Five day course of antibacterials for uncomplicated urinary infections. Urol. 8: 450 (1976).
15. R.N. Gruneberg, and W. Brumfitt. Single-dose treatment of acute urinary tract infection: a controlled trial. Br. Med. J. 3: 649 (1967).
16. L.S.T. Fang, N.E.T. Rubin and R. Rubin. Efficacy of single-dose and conventional amoxicillin therapy in UTI localized by the antibody-coated bacteria technique. N. Engl. J. Med. 298: 413 (1978).
17. G.K.M. Harding, F.J. Buckwald, T.J. Marrie, L. Thompson, R.B. Light and A.R. Ronald. Prophylaxis of recurrent urinary tract infection in female patients: Efficacy of low-dose thrice weekly therapy with trimethoprim-sulfamethoxazole. J.A.M.A. 242: 1975, Nov. 2 (1979).

## MURINE MODELS FOR STUDYING THE PATHOGENESIS AND TREATMENT OF PYELONEPHRITIS

Prabhavathi B. Fernandes, Nathan L. Shipkowitz, and Robert R. Bower

Pharmaceutical Products Division
Abbott Laboratories
North Chicago, Illinois

A variety of animal models have been used to study the pathogenesis and treatment of pyelonephritis in man. These models have employed a variety of animals such as monkeys, rabbits, guinea pigs, rats, and mice, and have been extensively reviewed by Cotran (1).

Experimental animals are remarkably resistant to urinary tract infections. Therefore, in most experimental models, the kidneys are damaged to ensure infection. Various methods of damaging the kidneys prior to infection have been used (1-7). Infection in the kidneys can also be promoted by ligation of the ureters to prevent urine flow (8) or by directly injecting large numbers of bacteria into the bladder of normal (9), water-diuresed (10), or hormone-treated animals (11).

In developing animal models, an attempt should be made to simulate human disease as closely as possible. To do this, it is necessary to understand host and bacterial factors and their interaction with each other (Table 1). These factors have been reviewed by Sobel and Kaye (8). The healthy host is one in which the physical and chemical conditions at the site of infection are inhospitable for the bacterium. In addition, the host actively defends itself against the bacterium with both the natural and acquired immune response. The bacterium, on the other hand, defends itself against the immune response of the host and adapts to the unnatural environment of the urinary tract.

### HOST FACTORS

Certain people are more prone to urinary tract infections than others, because host factors which normally prevent infection are changed in such a way as to allow bacteria to colonize the urinary tract. The mechanisms by which normal host factors prevent urinary tract infections are described in the following section. Physical factors, such as the flow of urine, prevent bacteria from gaining a foothold in the bladder. Obstruction of urine flow, such as that caused by anatomical abnormalities, stones, or foreign bodies such as catheters diminishes this host defense mechanism. The acidic pH and high osmolality of urine

Table 1. Host and Bacterial Factors Influencing the Pathogenesis of Urinary Tract Infections

| Host Factors | Bacterial Factors |
|---|---|
| 1. Flow of urine | 1. O antigen (LSP) |
| 2. Urea content of urine | 2. K antigen (capsule) |
| 3. $NH_3$ content of urine | 3. Serum resistance |
| 4. pH - Organic acids in urine, eg., hippuric and B-hydroxybutyric acid | 4. Adhesins (pili or fimbriae) - MS, MR, especially P adhesin |
| 5. Globoseries glycolipid and mannose receptors for MR and MS pili | 5. Flagella - chemotaxis |
| 6. Uromucoid | 6. Hemolysins |
| 7. Mucopolysacchride lining the bladder | 7. IgA proteases |
| 8. Normal flora - lactobacilli | |
| 9. Immunoglobulins, IgG, IgM and IgA | |
| 10. Cellular immunity - T lymphocytes - Macrophages and neutrophils | |

are also not conducive to bacterial growth (12). The high urea and ammonia concentrations in urine inhibit the growth of most bacteria except Proteus (8). Urea actually enhances the growth of the urea-splitting organism, Proteus. This has been shown by inhibiting Proteus infection in the urinary tract of mice by administering hydroxyurea and thiourea at the time of infection. These compounds inhibit the urease activity of Proteus and prevent the organism from infecting the urinary tract (13). Organic acids which are undissociated at the low pH of urine also inhibit bacterial growth (8). Other factors such as lysozyme, prostatic fluid, anti-B isohaemagglutinin, uromucoid (Tamm-Horsfall protein) and the normal flora made up of lactobacilli also play a role in defense against urinary tract infection (8). These defenses are compromised in certain disease states wherein the urinary tract is often infected. If bacteria overcome the physical and chemical defenses and reach the mucosa of the bladder, they have been shown to be efficiently cleared by a leukocyte response (14). The bladder epithelium is also protected by a mucopolysaccharide layer lining the area. This layer is presumed to interfere with adherence. If the bacteria succeed in persisting in the bladder, they can reach the kidneys via the ureters. In most situations, bacteria can survive and multiply in the medulla of the kidneys where the high osmolality and ammonia concentration prevent the activity of phagocytes and complement (15). The kidney cortex is less often infected because phagocytes, immune globulins, and complements are active at this site.

## BACTERIAL FACTORS

Escherichia coli is the bacterium most commonly isolated from urinary tract infections, but other organisms such as Proteus and Pseudomonas are also important pathogens at this site. E. coli isolated from the urinary tract usually belong to certain serotypes (16). These E. coli originate in the large bowel and colonize the periurethral area. The lipopolysaccharide (LPS) structure of these serotypes has been identified as an important virulence factor (17). The uropathogenic E. coli also have other virulence factors such as pili or fimbriae. There are at least two classes of pili: the mannose sensitive (MS or Type I) and mannose resistant (MR or Type X and P) pili (18). One type of MR pilus, the P adhesin, has been shown to play a major role in adherence (1920). MS pili bind to mannose receptors on many types of cells (21) including sheep red blood cells, thereby causing agglutination. These pili are probably important in periurethral and bladder colonization by *E. coli* because epithelial cells lining these areas have been found to be rich in mannose (22).

The importance of MS pili in adherence has been shown in experimental infection of mice. In mice, adherence to cells lining the urinary tract can be prevented by mixing *E. coli* with methyl- -D-mannopyranoside. In these studies, *Proteus mirabilis* strains were not inhibited by such treatment because MS pili are not used for adherence by this organism (22).

The ability of *E. coli* to adhere to mucous cell membranes is proposed to be essential for the initiation of urinary tract infection (23,25). Nephritogenic *E. coli* possess the P adhesins, which bind to α-D-Gal-p-(1 ⟶ 4) – β-D-GalP portion of glycosphinogolipid receptors on uroepithelial cells (26,27). Subjects with blood group p phenotype, a rare blood group, lack these receptors for nephritogenic *E. coli* (25) and are therefore less susceptible to urinary tract infection with *E. coli*. On the other hand, susceptibility to colonization has been linked to an increased representation of the $P_1$ blood group phenotype. Once the *E. coli* bearing MR and MS pili reach the kidneys they undergo phenotypic variation and lose their MS pili. This selective elimination of MS pili is of survival advantage to *E. coli* because phagocytes also bear mannose receptors on their surface. If the *E. coli* retained the MS pili, they would bind to phagocytes and be engulfed. Phagocytes do not have the globoseries of glycolipids which are receptors for P adhesins (19,28); therefore, the organisms are actually protected from phagocytosis by the P adhesins.

*E. coli* isolated from patients with asymptomatic bacteriuria or cystitis are generally serum sensitive (29). If however, these organisms find their way to the kidneys, they become serum resistant (11,30). Change to serum resistance is of survival advantage as the organisms cannot be lysed by serum complement. Many serum-resistant strains also possess the K antigen which is another adaptation which helps the bacteria to escape phagocytosis (31,32). The role of bacterial flagella and motility in infection has been less well studied. It is known that urine is a strong attractant for *E. coli* (33). Glucose and amino acids in urine appear to be the main chemoattractants. Thus bacterial chemotaxis towards urine may be a virulence factor.

Other virulence factors such as hemolysins may also be of advantage to the bacterium. Urinary isolates of *E. coli* are frequently hemolytic (34) and hemolytic *E. coli* are generally more virulent in animal models (35). In certain urinary isolates of *E. coli* the genes for hemolysin production (Hly) are closely linked to those for MR adhesins (35), but these genes were found to differ in different strains because they had restriction site heterogeneity. Therefore, Low and co-workers have suggested that the linkage between MR adhesin genes and Hly occurred more than once through independent events because such a linkage may have survival advantage (35). Hemolysin has also been implicated as a virulence factor in *Pseudomonas aeruginosa* strains which cause pyelonephritis (36).

In summary, virulence is not determined by any single virulence factor but by a combination of a number of contributing factors which have been described in this section.

IMMUNE RESPONSE TO INFECTION

An IgG, IgM, or IgA response is not generally observed if the infection is restricted to the lower urinary tract (37,32). However, after kidney infection, an IgG, IgM, and IgA response to O antigen is produced (38). IgM antibodies to K antigen are also produced (31,39,37). Antilipid A antibodies have also been detected in pyelonephritis (40). IgM antibodies have been shown to be important in protecting rats from urinary tract infection in an experimental model (37). Although no secretory IgA has been detected in a rat model, it is possible that an IgA response does occur but is undetectable because of the diluting effect of urine (40). It has been noted that local immunity at the mucosal surface resulting from either intravesicular (37) or oral (40) immunization is necessary to protect animals from ascending pyelonephritis. It is interesting that although IgA antibodies could not be detected in the urine of rats after oral immunization, it could be detected in the bronchial secretions (40). It is possible that gram negative bacteria, including E. coli, Proteus, and Pseudomonas produce IgA proteases in order to defend themselves against IgA antibodies in the urinary tract (41).

The genetic factors involved in susceptibility or resistance to urinary tract infection in man are unknown. This question has been recently examined by Svanborg-Eden and co-workers (42). Mouse strains with known deficiencies in the immune system were used to study the role of the immune response in rendering a host susceptible or resistant to pyelonephritis. Mice which showed a low mitogenic response to LPS, e.g., the C3H/HeJ ($LPS^d/LPS^d$) strain, were significantly more susceptible to pyelonephritis than their C3H/HeN ($LPS^n/LPS^n$) counterpart which showed a high mitogenic response to LPS. These mice are considered identical except for a genetic difference in the traits encoded for by the LPS gene. Strains of mice deficient in other aspects of the immune response such as T cells (nude mice) or macrophage response (A/J mice) were not more susceptible to renal infection than normal mice. Although the susceptibility to infection is unchanged in nude mice, the duration of infection has been found to be significantly longer (43). Therefore the cellular immune response may play a role in eradicating bacteria from the kidneys. It has also been observed that mice with macrophage deficiency (A/J strains) are more susceptible to bladder infection than normal mice (42). This finding supports the findings of Cobbs and Kaye (14) who showed a relationship between the clearance of bacteria and the migration of leukocytes within the bladder mucosa.

DESCRIPTION OF MURINE MODELS

Although animal models have been described in several animal species, only pyelonephritis models in mice will be described in the following section. Mice are preferred over rats because their uroepithelial cells possess globoseries glycolipid receptors for P pili which are similar to those found in man. The uroepithelial cells of rats do not have such receptors. E. coli is the best characterized urinary pathogen, therefore, most of this discussion will refer to E. coli with only occasional references to Proteus and Pseudomonas.

Two general methods are used to produce pyelonephritis in mice: 1) ascending infection in normal or diuresed mice, and 2) hematogenous infection of normal or damaged kidneys.

The ascending model for pyelonephritis in normal mice closely resembles the pathogenesis of the disease in man and involves no chemical or physical manipulation of the kidneys. This model has been described by Hagburg and co-workers (9). In this method, mice are forced to void by gently compressing the abdomen. They are then anesthetized with ether and a soft polyethylene catheter is inserted transurethrally into the urinary bladder. The catheter is fitted to a syringe and an inoculum of 0.05 ml of $10^{10}$ bacteria/ml is injected into the bladder. The catheter is then withdrawn. A large inoculum size is needed to obtain a reasonable level of infection. E. coli without P adhesins do not cause pyelonephritis in this model. Administration of analogues of globoseries glycolipids has been shown to inhibit the development of pyelonephritis using this model (44).

One frequently observed problem with this model is that only 50% of the infected mice may develop an infection. In addition, kidney infection levels vary considerably, the numbers of viable bacteria ranging from $10^2$ CFUs to $10^6$ CFUs two days after infection. This variation in the infection level and susceptibility to infection may be another indication that this is a realistic model for human pyelonephritis. However, for reliable tests of efficacy of antibacterial agents in animal models, the infection of the kidneys should be reproducible and at a high infection level of approximately $10^6$ CFUs. Drugs can then be evaluated on their ability to consistently reduce or clear the infection. A model for P. aeruginosa ascending pyelonephritis has been reported by Nishi and Tsuchiya (45). In this model, Pseudomonas was injected transurethrally with a syringe and the urethral meatus was clamped immediately after injection. By obstructing urine flow in this manner, a consistent infection was obtained in all animals. This model has been used successfully to evaluate new antibacterial agents (45).

Another ascending urinary tract infection model involves forced diuresis of mice prior to infection (46). This model is based upon the knowledge that the important natural defense mechanisms in the urinary tract are the high osmotic strength of urine and its high urea and ammonia concentrations, each of which is considerably reduced during diuresis. The specific gravity of urine is reduced from 1.03 in normal mice to 1.01 in diuresed mice. The pH of urine in diuresed mice is higher than in normal mice. The higher pH allows bacteria to grow in urine, adhere to the bladder epithelium, ascend the ureters, and infect the kidneys.

Female mice (CF-1, CD-1, and other strains are susceptible) are diuresed for 3-5 days with 5% glucose in water. The food intake of the diuresed mice is limited to 1 g of mouse chow per mouse per day. The mice are anesthetized with ether and a small mid-line abdominal incision is made. The bladder is exposed and 0.05 ml ($\sim 10^7$ CFU) of an 18 hour E. coli culture is injected into the bladder. The renal infection is maintained by continuing diuresis for as long as three months. The infection level in the kidneys is in the range of $10^3$-$10^7$ CFUs depending upon the strain used. Certain strains are more virulent than others and we found that some strains, possessing K antigen and hemolysin, become invasive and kill a large number of infected mice. Without diuresis, however, very few mice are infected and the infection level are low ($\sim 10^2$ CFUs). The histopathology of the kidneys of mice infected in this manner has been described previously (34). One week after infection histological lesions were seen in the renal pelvis. Four weeks after infection severe changes of pyelonephritis were seen including polymorphonuclear casts, necrotising abscesses, mononuclear infiltrate, tubular atrophy, and interstitial scarring. The infection generally goes not extend to the cortex and the organisms are restricted to the medulla.

Increased antibody titers have also been detected at four weeks after infection. This model has been useful in studying certain host defense factors such as the osmotic strength of urine. One drawback of the model is that the ability to cause infection in this model does not correllate with the presence of P adhesins on E. coli (47). Therefore, it is argued that the true pathogenesis of ascending pyelonephritis cannot be studied with this model.

The diuresed mouse model has been used successfully to evaluate new antibacterial agents (48). This model of pyelonephritis was used to evaluate the relative potencies of aztreonam, cefotaxime, and ampicillin against a β-lactamase producing strain of E. coli (P.B. Fernandes, D.P. Bonner, R.R. Whitney, B.H. Miller, C.O. Baugh, and R.B. Sykes. SQ 26, 776: Efficacy in experimental infections. Abst # 490 presented at the 21st Interscience Conference on Antimicrobial Agents and Chemotherapy, Nov. 4-6, 1981). Mice were treated by subcutaneous injections on the 7-10th day after infection. Three different dosage levels (25, 6.3, and 1.6 mg/kg/day) of aztreonam and cefotaxime were tested. Ampicillin was tested only at a dose of 100 mg/kg/day. Ten mice were used for each dosage level and the daily dose was administered as two injections spaced 6 hours apart. A group of ten mice was left untreated as controls for the infection. Mice were killed 18 hours after the last treatment and the kidneys were removed, homogenized in 5 ml of water, and cultured quantitatively. The geometric mean of the viable bacterial counts in the kidneys for each group of treated and untreated was then determined and the dose of antibacterial agent required to reduce the mean viable count by 99% of that found in the untreated group of mice was calculated. This was taken to be the effective dose of the antibacterial agent. The results are shown in Figure 1. A significant reduction in viable counts was obtained with aztreonam and cefotaxime. A good dose response was also noted with these β-lactams. Ampicillin had no effect on this strain of E. coli, showing that β-lactamase was produced in vivo and compounds like cefotaxime and aztreonam could be effective in urinary tract infections caused by such organisms. One of the disadvantages of this model for evaluation of the potency of antibacterial agents is that there is a wide range in the infection level of the untreated control animals. The kidneys of some animals are not infected. This poses a problem for statistical analysis because the median effective doses ($ED_{50}$) which can be calculated have wide confidence intervals.

## MODELS FOR HEMATOGENOUS INFECTION OF KIDNEYS

The kidneys can be infected by the hematogenous route after prior damage to the kidneys by injection of various chemicals or by mechanical injury to the kidneys. If normal mice are infected by the hematogenous route, it is difficult to establish a kidney infection (1). An acute suppurative infection of the kidneys can be caused by direct injection of bacteria into the kidneys (7). Although the hematogenous route of infection is unusual in man, this method has been used most frequently for the evaluation of antibiotics. These methods are generally simple to perform and the infection level in the kidneys are uniformly high.

Several methods to produce mechanical injury to the kidney have been described (1,49). These include renal massage (3) and ligation of the ureters (4). Chemicals such as 2-bromoethylamine hydrochloride (50) or carrageenan (51) have been used to produce renal damage in mice. Bromoethylamine hydrobromide (BEA) causes papillary necrosis when injected systemically (52). It is known to produce disseminated intravasular coagulation and deposits in the liver and kidneys (52). The dose of carrageenan used to induce renal damage in the pyelonephritis model has

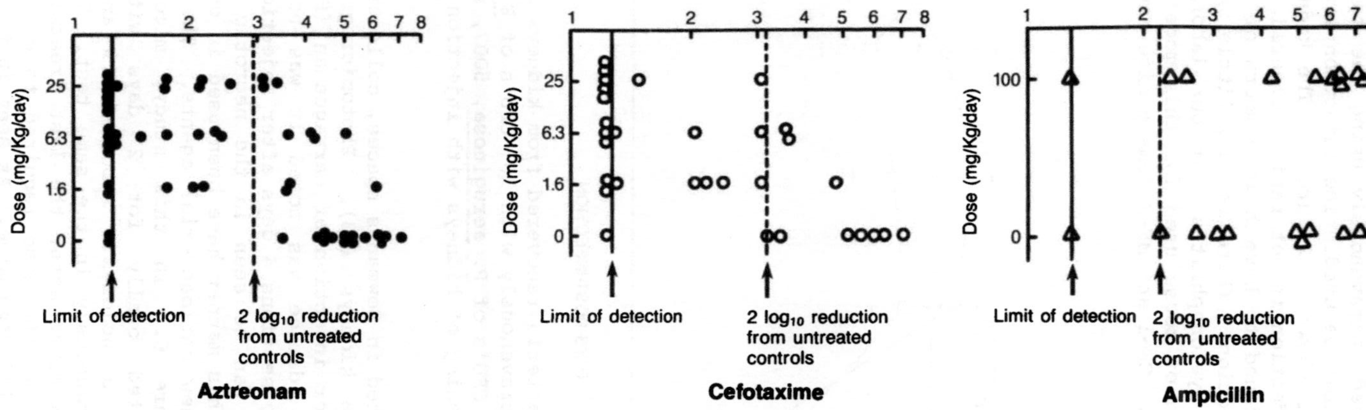


Fig. 1 Efficacy of aztreonam, cefotaxime, and ampicillin against E. coli (Sc 12, 199) in ascending urinary tract infection. The MIC of aztreonam, cefotaxime and ampicillin was <0.2, <0.3 and <50 mcg/ml, respectively. The mice were treated subcutaneously on the 7-10th day after infection. The $ED_{50}$ (median effective dose) calculated on the basis of a 99% reduction in viable counts ($Log_{10}$ CFUS in 2 kidneys) were: Aztreonam <1.6 mg/kg/day; cefotaxime <1.6 mg/kg/day; and ampicillin <100 mg/kg/day.

been adjusted so that few systemic effects are seen. The kidneys are "conditioned" by injecting 10 mg/kg in 0.2 ml of water intravenously in mice prior to injection of bacteria. Seven days after injection of carrageenan, 0.2 ml of an 18 hour culture diluted to contain approximately $10^5$ CFUs of E. coli 3100 or approximately $10^6$ CFUs of P. aeurginosa 5007, is injected intravenously using the tail vein. Other bacterial strains may possibly be used. The infection level with each of the two organisms tested is shown in Figure 2. The kidneys are consistently infected and the infection is not rapidly cleared. The kidneys of untreated mice have been found to have high numbers of bacteria for as long as 15 days after infection. There is very little mortality associated with this model for pyelonephritis. In our laboratories, it has been noted that the strain of mouse used for this model is critical to obtaining kidney infection. CF-1 and MF-2 female mice have been successfully used.

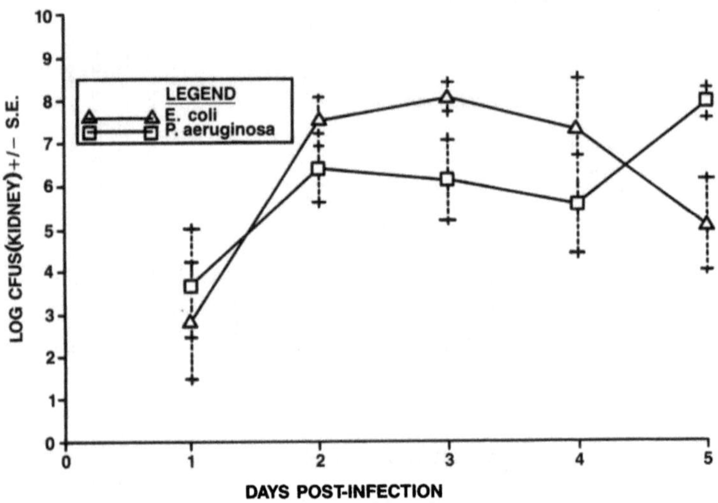


Fig. 2 Number of bacteria recovered from kidneys of mice injected intravenously with $10^5$ CFU's of E. coli, 3100 or $10^6$ CFU's of P. aeruginosa, 5007, following pre-conditioning of kidneys with injection of carrageenan.

Carrageenan is deposited in Bowman's spaces, collecting tubules, and medullary pyramids of the kidneys (53). Photomicrographs of kidney sections taken 7 days after injection of carrageenan (Figure 3a and b) show that although kidney damage was noted it was not overwhelming. Figures 4 and 5 show kidney sections 4 days after injection with E. coli. Large numbers of bacteria can be seen in the necrotic tubules (Figure 5a&b). Mice infected in this manner have been used in our laboratory to evaluate the potency of new antibacterial agents. The results of one study are shown in Figure 6. In this study, mice with E. coli pyelonephritis were treated orally for 2 days with amoxicillin, norfloxacin, and two new quinolones: Abbott-56619 and Abbott-56620. Gentamicin was used subcutaneously in the same test. The kidneys were cultured quantitatively 18 hours after the last treatment. The median effective dose was defined as the dose required to clear the infection from the kidneys of 50% of infected mice. As seen in the figure, the two new quinolones A-56619 and A-56620, were significantly more effective than norfloxacin and amoxicillin in treating this infection orally. They were also significantly better than gentamicin which was administered subcutaneously.

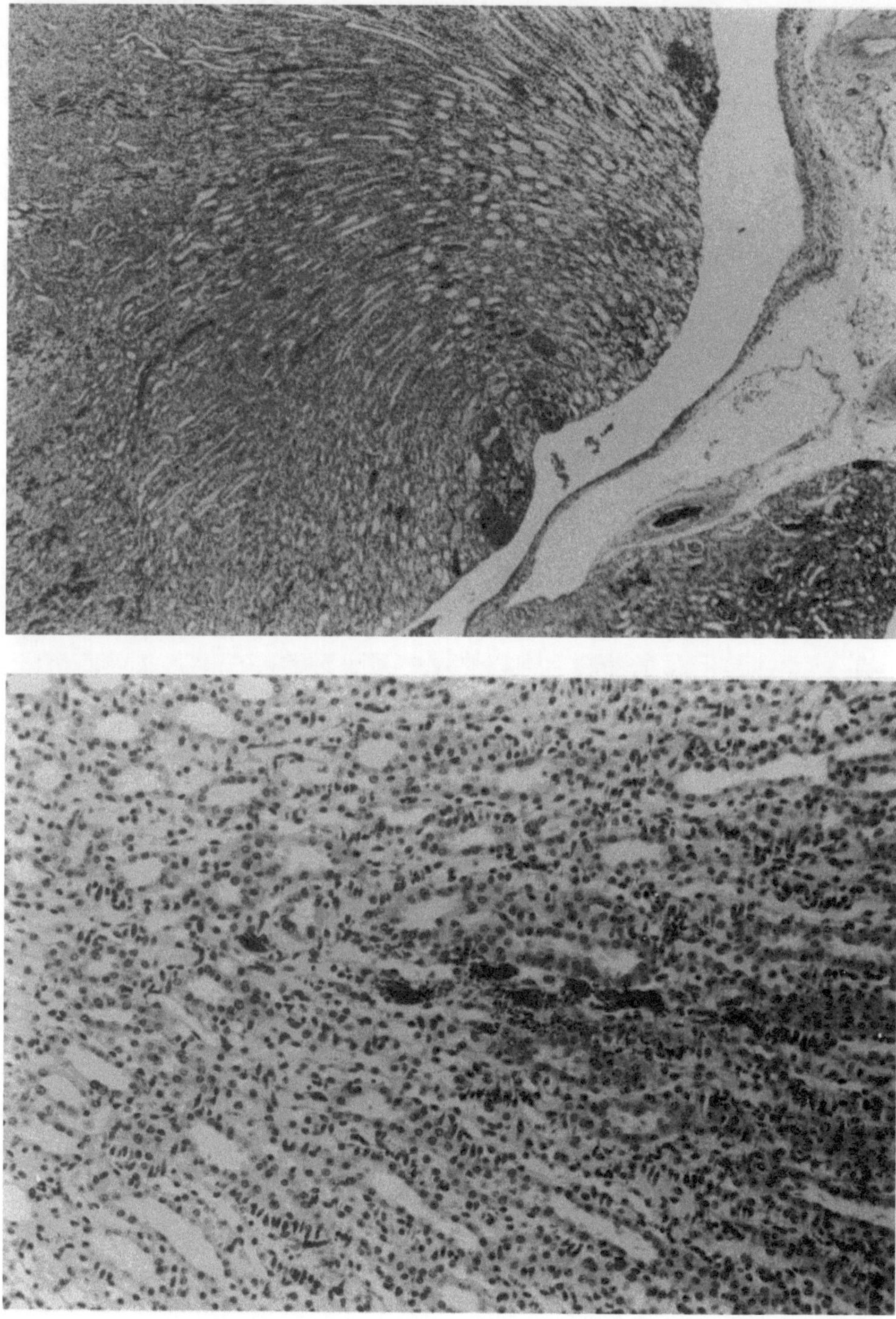

Fig. 3 Microscopic appearance of the renal medulla showing minimal focal cortical tubular dilatations and minimal focal cortical cell basophilia with and without proteinaceous casts. (Top = 39X; bottom = 63X).

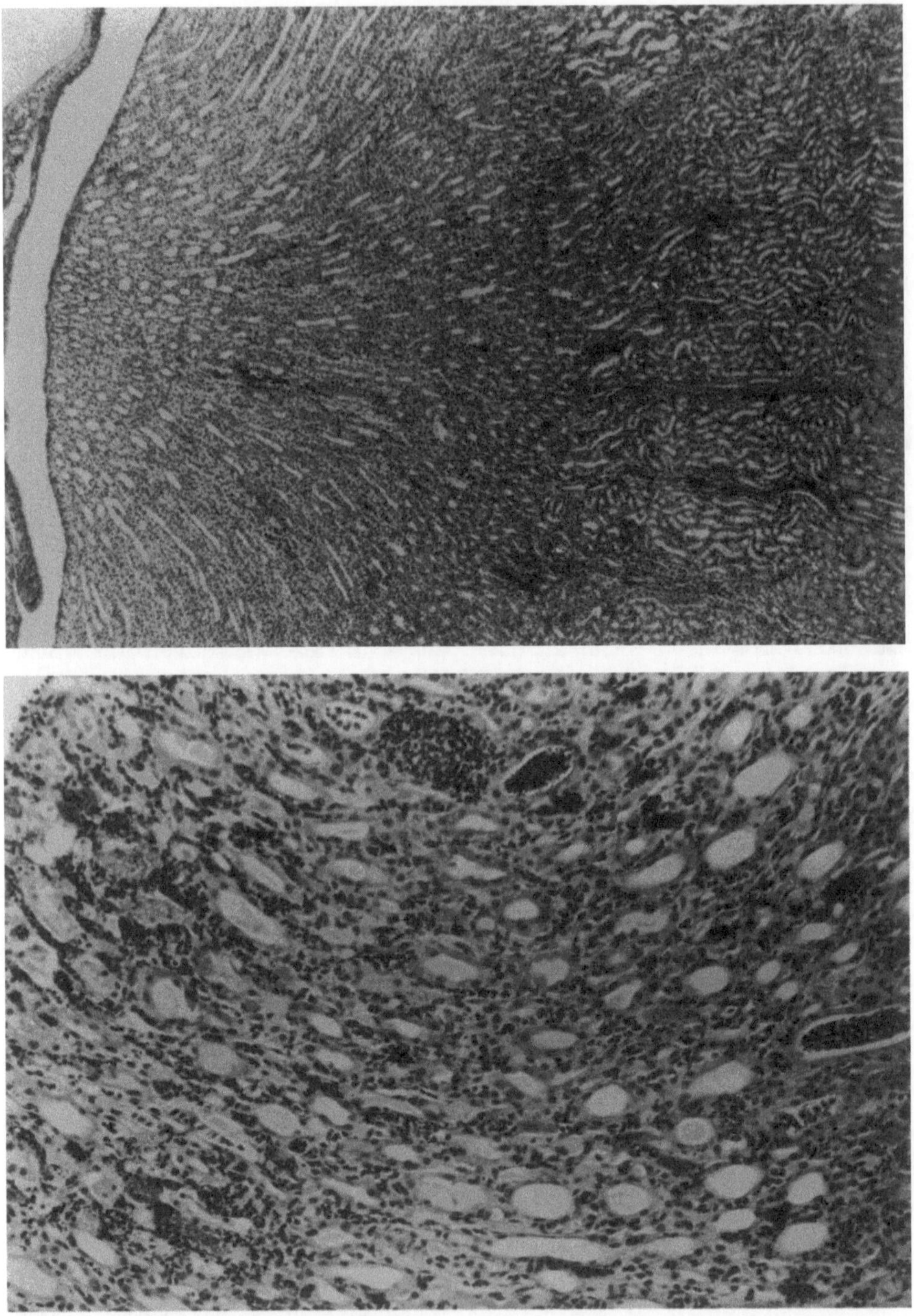

Fig. 4 Hematogenous pyelonephritis of carrageenan damaged kidneys. Microscopic appearance of the renal papilla showing various degrees of tubular necrosis with dilatation, tubular and intertubular inflammatory cell infiltration with hyperemia. (Top) A low magnification (haematoxylin and Eosin stain) (39X); (Bottom) Slightly higher magnification (63X).

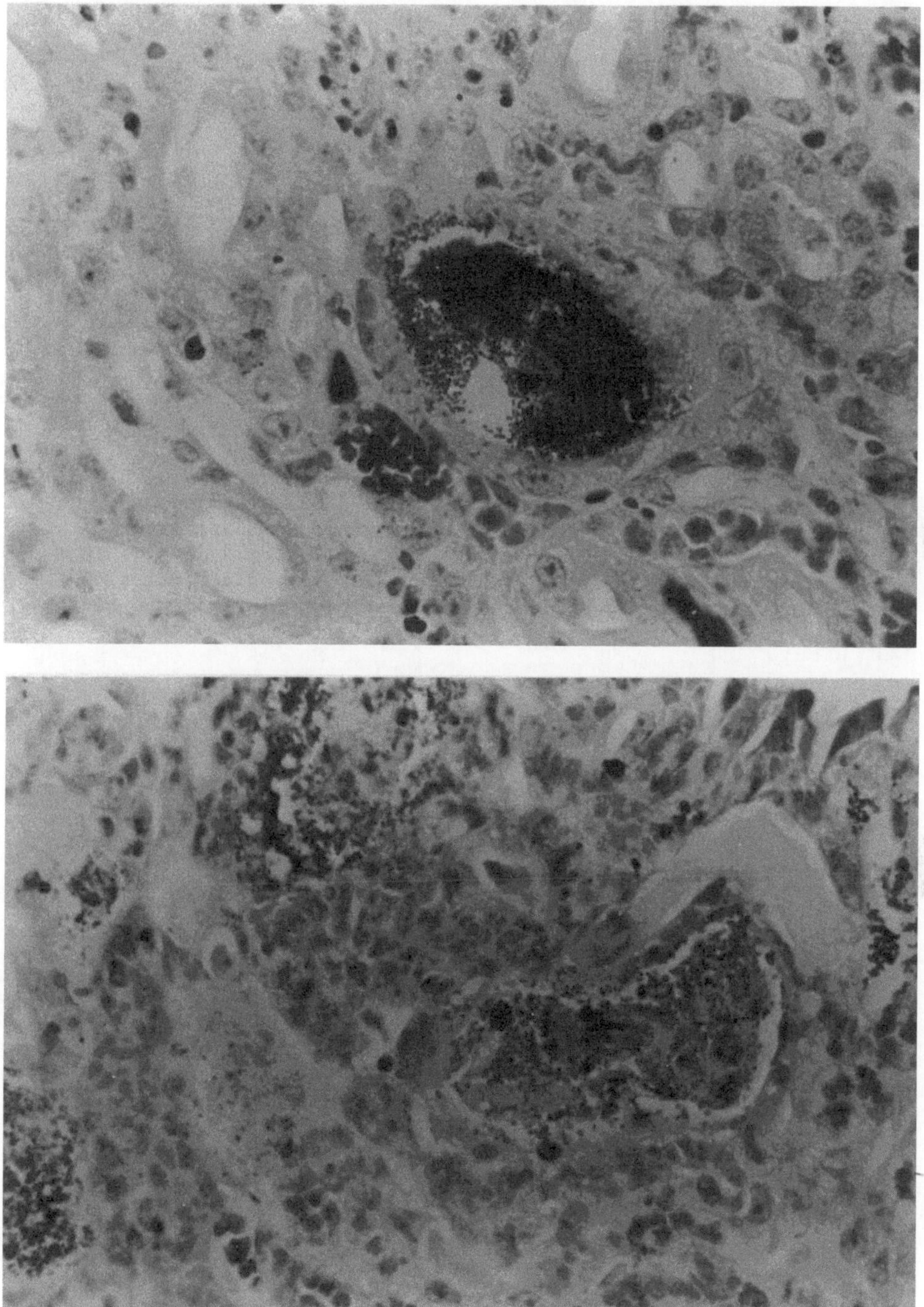

Fig. 5 Hematogenous pyelonephritis of carrageenan damaged kidney. Note the bacterial colonies in the necrotic tubules (Brown-Brenn stain). Top is 390X and Bottom is 625X.

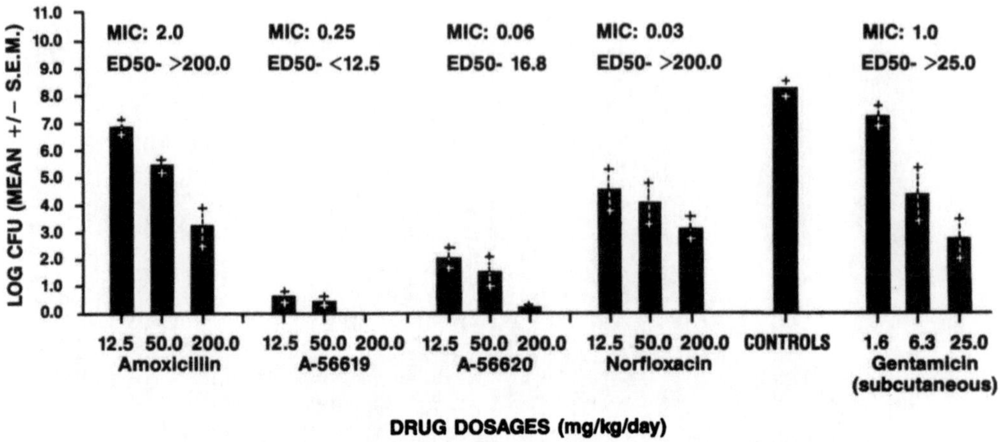


Fig. 6 Efficacy of quinolones used orally and gentamicin used subcutaneously in treating E. coli, 3100 hematogenous pyelonephritis. Treatment was started 24 hours after infection. The mice were treated orally for 2 days. MIC = minimum inhibitory concentration, $ED_{50}$ = median effective dose in mg/kg/day required to clear bacteria from the kidneys.

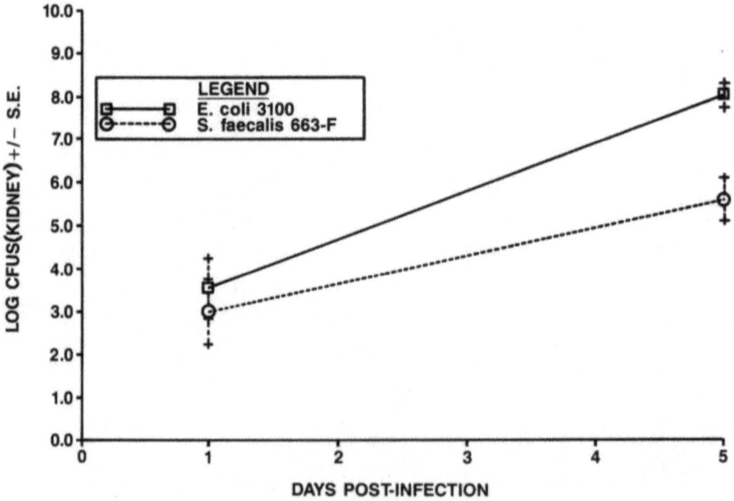


Fig. 7 Number of bacteria recovered from kidneys of mice infected with a mixture of E. coli 3100 and S. faecalis CMX 663F.

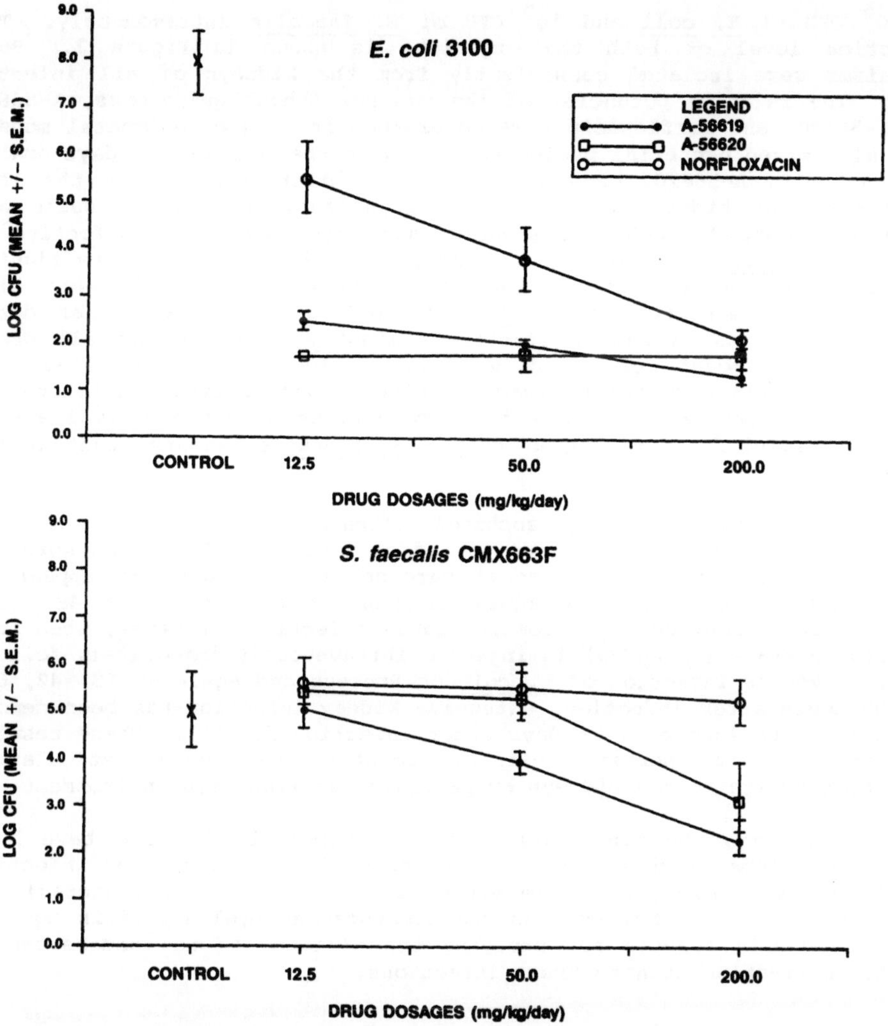


Fig. 8 Efficacy of quinolones in treating E. coli and S. 663F pyelonepritis in hematogenous pyelonephritis in mice. The MIC of norfloxacin, A-56619 and a-56620 against E. coli 3100 was 0.03, 0.25 and 0.06 ug/ml, respectively. The MIC of norfloxacin, A-56619 and A-56620 against S. faecalis CMX 663F was 4, 8 and 4 ug/ml, respectively. Treatment was started 24 hr after infection and the mice were treated orally for 3 days.

Streptococcus faecalis is frequently isolated along with E. coli from urinary tract infections. After eradication of E. coli, enterococcal overgrowth of the urinary tract has been reported (54). In order to evaluate new antibacterial agents in mixed infections, we have developed a pyelonephritis model in mice using a mixture of E. coli 3100 and S. faecalis CMX 663F. Carrageenan treated mice were infected with a mixture of $10^5$ CFU of E. coli and $10^5$ CFU of S. faecalis intravenously. The infection level of both the organisms is shown in Figure 7. Both organisms were isolated consistently from the kidneys of all infected mice. The relative potencies of the two new Abbott quinolones, A-56619 and A-56620, and norfloxacin were determined in this experimental model. Mice with mixed bacterial pyelonephritis were treated for two days orally with A-56619, A-56620, or norfloxacin. Eighteen hours after the last treatment, the kidneys were cultured quantitatively. The results are shown in Figure 8. A-56619, A-56620, and norfloxacin were effective in treating E. coli in the mixed infection; A-56619 and A-56620 were significantly more potent than norfloxacin. A-56619 and A-56620 were also effective in reducing the S. faecalis infection at the higher doses tested. Norfloxacin was ineffective against S. faecalis at all doses tested. This model for mixed bacterial pyelonephritis should also be useful in determining the efficacy of other broad spectrum antibacterial agents or to determine if selected combinations of antibacterial agents could be useful for treating E. coli - S. faecalis urinary tract infections.

Another chemical, iron sorbitol citrate has also been used to "condition" the kidneys in order to induce infection(55). Iron sorbitol citrate is deposited in the renal parenchyma, but does not appear to damage renal tissue because administration of the iron salt 48 hours prior to infection does not promote kidney infection. However, when iron sorbitol citrate (30 mg/kg) is injected intravenously immediately following intravenous injection of E. coli or Proteus and again at 18, 42, 66, and 90 hours after infection, extensive kidney infection has been demonstrated for as long as 7-14 days after infection (56,55). These results suggest that iron sorbitol citrate promotes infection by stimulating bacterial growth in the kidneys by providing an iron rich environment.

In summary, various models for pyelonephritis in mice have been described. Some of these, such as the ascending urinary tract infecting model in normal mice, are more useful for studying the pathogenesis of pyelonephritis. Others, such as the hematogenous pyelonephritis models, are more easily adapted for studying the efficacy of new antibacterial agents in treating urinary tract infections.

ACKNOWLEDGEMENT

We thank Joan Doerr and Cynthia David for typing this manuscript. We also appreciate the cooperation of Dr. Sait Tekeli who provided us with the histopathology photographs. We also thank John Stamm for his editorial assistance. Figure 8 was provided by Dr. Sanathanan from the Abbott Laboratories Biostatistics Department.

REFERENCES

1. R.S. Cotran. Experimental pyelonephritis, in: "The Kidney: Morphology, Biochemistry, Physiology", C. Roullier, A.F. Muller, ed. Vol. II. Academic Press, New York (1969).
2. C.P. Adler, H. Ritzman, and H.U. Zollinger, Vergleichende untersuchungen uber die hamatogene und die ascendierende pyelonephritis bei ratten, Virchows Arch [Pathol Anat]: 347: 277 (1969).
3. A.I. Baude, A.P. Shapiro, and J. Siemienski, Hematogenous pyelonephritis in rats III. Relationship of bacterial species to the pathogenesis of acute pyelonephritis, J. Bacterial. 77: 270 (1959).
4. R.S. Cotran E., Vivaldi, D.P., Zangwill, and E.H. Kass, Retrograde

Proteus pyelonephritis in rats, Bacteriologic, pathologic, and fluorescent-antibody studies, Am. J. Pathol. 43: 1 (1963).
5. R.H. Heptinstall. Experimental pyelonephritis. Bacteriological and morphological studies on the ascending route of infection in the rat, Nephron. 1: 73 (1964).
6. B.W. Hunter, L.L., Souda, and J.P. Sanford. Antibiotic therapy in established chronic experimental Proteus mirabilis pyelonephritis, Antimicrob. Agents Chemother. 3: 608 (1963).
7. T.E. Miller, and K.B. Robinson. Experimental pyelonephritis: a new method for inducing pyelonephritis in the rat, J. Infect. Dis. 127: 307 (1973).
8. J.D. Sobel, and D. Kaye. Host factors in the pathogenesis of urinary tract infections, Am. J. Med. 76: 122 (1984).
9. L. Hagberg, I. Engberg, R. Freter, J. Lam, S. Olling, and C. Svanborg-Eden. Ascending, unobstructed urinary tract infection in mice caused by pyelonephritogenic Escherichia coli of human origin, Infect. Immun. 40: 273 (1983).
10. L.R. Freedman. Experimental pyelonephritis XIII. On the ability of water diuresis to induce susceptibility to E. coli bacteriuria in the normal rat, Yale J. Biol. Med. 39: 255 (1967).
11. W. Henkel, and R., Commichau. Serumresistenz und nephropathogenitar antigenetisch difinierter Stamme von E. coli III, Experimentelle pyelonephritis mit unterschiedlick serum-resistenten keimen, Z. med. Mikrobiol. Immunol. 156: 297 (1971).
12. D. Kaye. Antibacterial activity of human urine, J. Clin. Invest. 47: 2374 (1968).
13. M. Aronson, O. Medalia and B. Griffel. Prevention of ascending pyelonephritis in mice by urease inhibitors, Nephron 12: 94 (1974).
14. C.G. Cobbs, and D., Kaye. Antibacterial mechanisms in the urinary bladder, Yale J. Biol. Med. 40: 93 (1967).
15. P.B. Beeson, and D. Rowley. The anticomplementary effect of kidney tissue, Its association with ammonia production, J. Exp. Med. 110: 685 (1959).
16. R.N. Gruneberg, D.A. Leigh, and W. Brumfitt. Escherichiau coli serotypes in urinary tract infection, in: Studies in domicillary antenatal and hospital practice in urinary tract infections," F. O'Grady and W. Brumfitt, ed., Oxford University Press, London (1968).
17. B. Kusecek, H. Wloch, A. Mercer, V. Vaisanen, G. Pluschke, T. Korhonen, and M. Achtman. Lipopolysaccharide, capsule, and fimbriae as virulence factors among 01, 07, 016, 018, 04 075 and K1, K5, or K100 Escherichia coli, Infect. Immun. 43: 368 (1984).
18. J.F. Van der Bosch, U. Verboom-Sohmer, P. Postma, J. DeGraaff and D. MacLaren, Mannose-sensitive and Mannose-resistant adherence to human uroepithelial cells and urinary virulence of Escherichia coli, Infect. Immun. 29: 226 (1980).
19. L. Hagberg, U. Jodal, T.K. Korhonen, G. Lidin-Janson, U. Lindberg, and C. Svanborg-Eden. Adhesion, hemagglutination, and virulence of Escherichia coli causing urinary tract infections, Infect. Immun. 31: 564 (1981).
20. C. Svanborg-Eden, B. Eriksson, and L.A. Hanson. Adhesion of Escherichia coli to human uroepithelial cells in vitro, Infect. Immun. 18: 767 (1977).
21. I. Ofek, A. Mosek, and N. Sharon. Mannose-specific adherence of Escherichia coli freshly excreted in the urine of patients with urinary tract infections, and of isolates subcultured from the infected urine, Infect. Immun. 34: 708 (1981).
22. M. Aronson, O. Medalia, L. Schori, D. Mirelman, N. Sharon, and I. Ofek. Prevention of colonization of the urinary tract of mice with Escherichia coli by blocking of bacterial adherence with methyl -D-mannopyranoide, J. Infect. Dis. 139: 329 (1979).

23. L. Hagberg, R. Hull, S. Hull, S. Falkow, R. Freter, and C. Svanborg-Eden. Contribution of adhesion to bacterial persistence in the mouse urinary tract, Infect. Immun. 40: 265 (1983).
24. C. Svanborg-Eden, R. Freter, L. Hagberg, R. Hull, S. Hull, H. Leffler, G. Schoolnik. Inhibition of experimental ascending urinary tract infection by an epithelial cell-surface receptor analogue, Nature (London) 298: 560 (1982).
25. Varsanen, V., L.G. Tallgren, P.H. Makela, G. Kallenius, H. Hultberg, J. Elo, A. Siitonen, C. Svanborg-Eden, S.B. Svenson, and T. Korhonen, Mannose-resistant haemagglutination and P antigen recognition are characteristic of Escherichia coli causing primary pyelonephritis, Lancet. II: 1366 (1981).
26. G. Kallenus, R. Mollby, H. Hultberg, S.B. Svenson, B. Cedergren, and J. Winberg, 1981. Structure of carbohydrate part of receptor on human uroepithelial cells for pyelonephritogenic Escherichia coli, Lancet II: 604 (1981).
27. H. Leffler, and C. Svanborg-Eden. Chemical identification of a glycospingolipid receptor for Escherichia coli attaching to human urinary tract epithelial cells and agglutinating human erythrocytes, FEMS Microbiol. Lett. 8: 127 (1980).
28. C. Svanborg-Eden, L.M. Bjursten, R. Hull, S. Hull, K.E. Magnusson, Z. Moldovano, and H. Leffler. Influence of adhesin on the interaction of Escherichia coli with human phagocytes, Infect. Immun. 44: 672 (1984).
29. U.L. Lindberg, A. Hanson, U. Jodal, G. Lidin-Janson, K. Lincoln, and S. Olling. Asymptomatic bacteriurea in school girls, II. Differences in Escherichia coli causing asymptomatic bacteriuria, Acta. Paediatr. Scand. 64: 432 (1975).
30. S. Olling, L.A. Hanson, J. Holmgen, U. Jodel, K. Lincoln and U. Lindberg. The bactericidal effect of normal human serum on E. coli strains from animals and from patients with urinary tract infections, Infection 1: 24 (1973).
31. A. Glynn, A. Brumfitt, and C.J. Howard. K antigens of Escherichia coli and renal involvement in urinary tract infections, Lancet 1: 514 (1971).
32. J.W. Smith, and B. Kaijser. The local immune response to Escherichia coli O and K antigen in experimental pyelonephritis, J. Clin. Invest. 58: 276 (1976).
33. B. Herrmann, and L.G. Burman. Chemoattracting effect of human urine on motile Escherichia coli, FEMS Microbiol. Lett. 20: 411 (1983).
34. G.M. Kalmanson, M. Turck, H.J. Harwick, and L.B. Guze. Urinary tract infection: Localization and virulence of Escherichia coli, Lancet 1: 134 (1975).
35. D. Low, V. David, D. Lark, G. Schoolnik, and S. Falkow. Gene cluster governing the production of hemolysin and mannose-resistant hemaglutination are closely linked in Escherichia coli serotype O4 and O6 isolates from urinary tract infections, Infect. Immun. 43: 353 (1984).
36. R.M. Al-Ssum, and D.M. Harris. The contribution of diffusable toxins of Pseudomonas aeruginosa to the pathogenesis of experimental pyelonephritis, J. Infect. 4: 49 (1982).
37. B. Kaijser, P. Larsson, and S. Olling. Protection against ascending Escherichia coli pyelonephritis in rats and significance of local immunity, Infect. Immun. 20: 78 (1978).
38. J.P. Sanford, B.W. Hunter, and L.L. Souda. The role of immunity in the pathogenesis of experimental hematogenous pyelonephritis, J. Exp. Med. 115: 383 (1962)
39. B. Kaijser. Immunology of Escherichia coli: K antigen and its relation to urinary tract infection, J. Infect. Dis. 127: 670 (1973).

40. I. Mattsby-Baltzer, L.A. Hanson, S. Olling, and B. Kaijser. Experimental Escherichia coli ascending pyelonephritis in rats: Active peroral immunization with live Escherichia coli, Infect. Immun. 35: 647 (1982).
41. F.H. Millazo, and G.J. Delisle. Immunoglobulin A proteases in gram-negative bacteria isolated from human urinary tract infections, Infect. Immun. 43: 11 (1984).
42. C. Svanborg-Eden, D. Briles, L. Hagberg, J. McGhee, and S. Michalec. Genetic factors in host resistance to urinary tract infection, Infection 12: 118 (1984).
43. H. Pitchon, R. Glassock, G.M. Kalmanson, and L.B. Guze. Experimental pyelonephritis: The effect of T-cell deficiency in the course of hematogenous enterococcal pyelonephritis in the mouse, Am. J. Pathol. 115: 25 (1984).
44. C. Svanborg-Eden, B. Andersson, L. Hagberg, L.A. Hanson, H. Lomberg, H. Leffler, G. Magnusson, G. Noori, J. Dahmen, and T. Sonderstrom. Receptor analogues and anti-pili antibodies as inhibitors of bacterial attachment in vivo and in vitro, Proc. N.Y. Acad. Sci. 409: 580 (1983).
45. T. Nishi, and K. Tsuchiya. Experimental urinary tract infection with Pseudomnonas aeruginosa in mice, Infect. Immun. 22: 508 (1978).
46. W.F. Keane, and L.R. Freedman. Experimental pyelonephritis XIV. Pyelonephritis in normal mice produced by inoculation of E. coli into the bladder lumen during water diuresis, Yale J. Biol. Med. 40: 231 (1967).
47. L.B. Guze, F. Silverblatt, J.Z. Montogomerie, K. Ishida, and G.M. Kalmanson. Lack of significance of pili in ascending Escherichia coli pyelonephritis, Scand. J. Infec. Dis. 15: 57 (1983).
48. E.G. Hubert, G.M. Kalmanson and L.B. Guze. Antibiotic therapy of Escherichia coli pyelonephritis produced in mice undergoing chronic diuresis, Antimicrob. Agents. Chemother. 8: 507 (1968).
49. M. Rocha, and F.R. Fekety. Acute inflammation in the renal cortex and medulla following thermal injury, J. Exp. Med. 119: 131 (1964).
50. E.H. Thiele. An in vivo pyelonephritis assay for screening therapeutic agents, J. Antibiot. 27: 31 (1984).
51. O. Zak, F. Kradolfer, E.A. Konopka, S. Kunz and E. Batt. CGP7174/E (Takeda SCE 129), Activity against systemic and urinary tract infections in mice and rats, in "Current Chemotherapy", Vol 2. Proceedings of the 19th International Congress of Chemotherapy, Zurich, ASM, Washington, D.C. 846 (1978).
52. A.Q. Thomson, and E.F. Fowler, Carrageenan: A review of its effects on the immune system, Agents and Actions 11 (3): 265 (1981).
53. E.F. Fowler, J.G. Simpson and A.W. Thomson. Histological and ultrastructural changes following carageenan injection in the mouse, J. Path. 132: 63 (1980).
54. R. Moellering. Enterococcal infections in patients treated with moxalactam, Rev. Infect. Dis. 4: S708 (1982).
55. J. Fletcher, and E. Goldstein. The effect of parenteral iron preparations on experimental pyelonephritis, Br. J. Exp. Pathol. 51: 280 (1970).
56. K.R. Comber. Pathogenesis of an experimental pyelonephritis model in the mouse and its use in the evaluation of antibiotics, in: "Chemotherapy", Vol 2, J.D., Williams and A.M. Gedes, ed., Plenum Publishing Corp., New York (1976).

# UROPATHOGENIC ESCHERICHIA COLI: MOLECULAR MECHANISMS OF ADHERENCE

Gary K. Schoolnik, Peter O'Hanley, David Lark,
Staffan Normark, Kenneth Vosti, and Stanley Falkow

From the Medical Service, Palo Alto Veterans
Administration Medical Center, and the Departments
of Medicine and Medical Microbiology, Stanford
University School of Medicine, Stanford, California

Escherichia coli isolated from endogenous infections of the urinary tract usually originate in the colon (1-3). From the stool, uropathogenic strains colonize the vaginal introitus and periurethral region (4). Colonization of uroepithelium may ensue, leading to bacteriuria. Symptoms arise when invasion of mucosa, cell death, and inflammation occur in the bladder or kidney. Therefore, cystitis and pyelonephritis may be viewed as the culmination of a sequence of events mediated by specific determinants of microbial virulence. It follows that uropathogenic E. coli are not simply the most prevalent fecal stains. Instead, they appear to manifest a pathogenic phenotype: they usually belong to a restricted number of O and K antigen serogroups (3-5); they are resistant to the bactericidal action of normal human serum (6-8); they secrete hemolysin (9-11), produce colicin V (12-13), and ferment salicin (14); and they attach to uroepithelial cells in vitro (15-17).

Colonization of the mucosa is the in vivo equivalent of epithelial cell adherence and a necessary precondition for bacteriuria, cystitis, and pyelonephritis. It is mediated by bacterial adhesions and the epithelial cell surface molecules to which they bind. The molecular basis for this phenomenon is the subject of this report.

ADHESIONS OF UROPATHOGENIC E. COLI

Most E. coli strains possess nonflagellar, proteinaceous appendages termed pili (or fimbriae) that serve to bind the bacteria to each other and to a variety of plant and animal cell surfaces. Two major classes of chromosomally encoded pili have been defined functionally by their receptor specificities. Type 1, or common pili, are termed mannose-sensitive. They bind Tamm-Horsfall uromucoid (18) (a mannose containing glycoprotein in the urine of placental animals), attach to African green monkey kidney cells (19), and their agglutination of guinea pig erythrocytes is inhibited by D-mannose and methyl- -D-mannopyranoside (20). Most human pyelonephritis E. coli isolates also express mannose-resistant pili, which bind neutral glycolipids of the globoseries including globotetraosylceramide and trihexosylceramide. These can be extracted from human uroepithelial cells (vida infra) and are antigens of the human P blood group system (21-22). They contain D-Gal p 1 4D-Gal p 1 and a synthetic analog of this disaccharide (Syn Gal-Gal) inhibits hemagglutination (23). Mannose-resistant pili with this binding specificity have been termed P fimbriae, Pap (pyelonephritis associated) pili, and Gal-Gal pili. Mannose-resistant pyelonephritogenic E. coli strains have also been identified that agglutinate human erythrocytes in the presence of mannose and Syn Gal-Gal (24). This property may be conferred by "X" pili (24) or by a nonpilus hemmaglutinin (25).

The relative prevalence of mannose-sensitive, mannose-resistant, and X pili expressed by strains of E. coli isolated from the feces of normal volunteers and from the urine of adult women with anatomically normal urinary tracts was assessed by hemagglutination, hapten inhibition of hemagglutination by carbohydrate receptor analogs, and carbohydrate-adsorbed latex agglutination assays. All isolates (Table 1) expressed mannose-sensitive pili. Gal-Gal pili were expressed by all pyelonephritis isolates, by 24 of 47 (51%) cystitis isolates, and by only 17 of 46 (40%) fecal isolates. X pili were expressed by four of nine (44%) pyelonephritis strains, 13 of 47 (28%) cystitis strains, and only 4 of 46 (9%) fecal isolates. These data are in general agreement with the reported incidence of Gal-Gal piliated E. coli in children with urinary tract infections. Kallenius *et al.* (26) detected Gal-Gal pili in 32 of 35 (91%) pyelonephritis isolates, 5 of 26 (19%) cystitis isolates, 5 of 36 (14%) strains in patients with asymptomatic bacteriuria and 6 of 82 (7%) strains isolated from the feces of healthy children.

Table 1. Pilus Receptor Specificity of Uropathogenic Escherichia coli

| Clinical Syndrome | Patient Group | % Pilus Receptor Specificity Gal-Gal | Mannose | X |
|---|---|---|---|---|
| Pyelonephritis | Adult | 100 | 100 | 44 |
| Cystitis | Adult | 51 | 100 | 28 |
| Normal Fecal Isolates | Adult | 40 | 100 | 9 |

These studies indicate that mannose-sensitive and Gal-Gal pili are simultaneously expressed by most pyelonephritic isolates, but they do not address their pathogenic significance. Molecular cloning of putative virulence determinants and the use of the recombinants in appropriate animal models of human disease can provide convincing evidence of their role in pathogenesis. This strategy was pursued by Hull *et al.* (27) who cloned, from a human pyelonephritis E. coli isolate, two distinct chromosomal fragments that separately encode mannose-sensitive or Gal-Gal pili. When harbored in a nonpiliated derivative of E. coli, K-12, the two recombinant plasmids were found to express either the mannose-resistant or the mannose-sensitive adherence property of the clinical isolate. The parent strain, the two recombinants, and the nonpiliated E. coli recipient were employed in a urinary tract infection model.

The prerequisites of a valid urinary tract infection model are as follows: (1) it must stimulate an ascending infection mode; (2) it should not entail obstruction to urine flow or traumatic manipulation of tissue; and (3) uroepithelial surfaces should exhibit, qualitatively and quantitatively, the same pilus receptors as those in man. Although many urinary tract infection models have been proposed (28), the 16 week Balb/c mouse was selected for these studies because its immune system is mature and the bladder epithelial cells of this species reportedly contain globotetraosylceramide and bind Gal-Gal pili (29).

Table II. Immunoperoxidase Detection of Syn Man-Man and Syn Gal-Gal Pilus Receptors in BALB/c Mouse Urogenital Tissue

| Tissue/Cell | Intensity of Pilus Disaccharide Receptor* | |
|---|---|---|
| | Syn Man-Man ‡ | Syn Gal-Gal§ |
| 1. Vagina | | |
| Squamous Epithelium | +3 | +3 |
| 2. Bladder | | |
| Transitional Epithelium | +3 | +2 |
| Lamina Propria ‖ | | |
| Fibroblasts | 0 | 0 |
| Smooth Muscle | +2 | +2 |
| 3. Ureter | | |
| Transitional Epithelium | +3 | +2 |
| 4. Renal Pelvis | | |
| Transitional Epithelium | +3 | +2 |
| 5. Kidney | | |
| Glomerulus | 0 | 0 |
| Proximal Tubulur Cells | +2 | +2 |
| Loop of Henle Cells | +1 | 0/+1 |
| Collecting Ducts | +3 | +3 |

* Intensity of pilus disaccharide receptor-graded 3+ (intense brown) to 0 (no brown reaction product).

‡ Mannose pilus receptor was assessed by monospecific, affinity-purified rabbit antibody to synthetic αD-Man (1→ 2)αD Man.

§ Gal-Gal pilus receptor was assessed by monospecific, affinity-purified rabbit antibody to synthetic αD-Gal (1→ 2)αD-Gal.

‖ The distribution of pilus receptors in the lamina propria of the bladder were the same throughout the urogenital tract.

The distribution of pilus receptor compounds on the genitourinary epithelial surfaces of the Balb/c mouse and man was assessed in greater detail to determine the model's validity (D. Lark, P. O'Hanley, D. Baker, F. Weinstein, and G. Schoolnik, unpublished observation). An avidin-biotin peroxidase immunohistochemical assay was performed with monospecific antibodies to the synthetic receptor analogs D-gal p 1 4D-Gal p and D-Man p 1 2D-Man p (Chemibiomed Limited, Edmonton, Alberta, Canada) for Gal-Gal and mannose-sensitive pili, respectively. The Gal-Gal pilus receptor analog was detected in all the indicated genitourinary tissues of both species (Table II) except the glomerulus and the loop of Henle. Its presence in vaginal epithelium may explain why vaginal colonization often precedes bacteriuria (4). Similarly, the concentration of the Gal-Gal pilus receptor analog in renal collecting ducts may account for the prevalence of Gal-Gal pili among pyelonephritogenic strains.

Pilus receptor carbohydrates were also sought in the urine of man and the Balb/c mouse. The urine of both species contains a titratable factor that inhibits the binding of mannose-sensitive pili to the receptor analog (P. O'Hanley, D. Lark, S. Falkow, and G. Schoolnik, unpublished observation). This factor was determined to be physically, chemically, and immunologically identical to the Tamm-Horsfall glycoprotein (30), which is produced by the ascending limb of the loop of Henle and the distal convoluted tubule and released into tubular urine. Also termed urinary slime, it may entrap mannose-sensitive piliated E. coli (18) and nullify their capacity to bind cell surface receptor carbohydrates. In contrast, no urine factor blocked the receptor-binding capacity of Gal-Gal pili.

Table III. Functional, Serologic and Chemical Properties of Escherichia coli Strains and Isolated Pili

| | | | | Agglutinating properties | | | |
|---|---|---|---|---|---|---|---|
| | | | | RBC Species | | Carbohydrate binding§ | |
| Strain | Pilus operon | Source | Antibiotic resistance | Human HA*/HAI‡ | Guinea Pig HA/HAI | Syn Gal-Gal | Syn Man-Man |
| J96 | MS+ Gal-Gal | Human pyelonephritis | None | +/Syn Gal-Gal | +/ αMM | + | + |
| SH48 | MS | Recombinant(J96 DNA) | Tetracycline | -/- | +/ αMM | - | + |
| HU849 | Gal-Gal | Recombinant(J96 DNA) | Chloramphenicol | +/Syn Gal-Gal | -/- | + | - |
| P678-54 | None | K12 derived host | None | -/- | -/- | - | - |
| Pili | N-terminal Sequence‖ (1 ... 25) | | Shared antigenicity¶ | | | | |
| SH48 | APTIPQGQGKVTFNGTVVDAPCSIS | | <5% | -/- | +/ αMM | - | + |
| HU849 | AATTVNGGTVHFKGEVVNAACAVD | | <5% | +/Syn Gal-Gal | -/- | + | - |

* Hemagglutination of human or guinea pig erythrocytes: +positive; -negative.

‡ Hapten inhibition of hemagglutination by Syn Gal-Gal or αMM ( αmethyl-mannoside) according to the method of O'Hanley et al. (13).

§ Agglutination of latex beads adsorbed with Syn Gal-Gal or Syn Man-Man (13): +positive; -negative.

‖ After O'Hanley et al. (13). Underlined residues are conserved.

¶ Determined by a two-step competitive ELISA (13).

The Balb/c mouse model was examined with four E. coli strains to assess the pathogenic significance of mannose-sensitive and Gal-Gal pili (23,31). Their binding properties are indicated in Table III. J96 is a pyelonephritis isolate that simultaneously expresses Gal-Gal and mannose-sensitive pili and is also hemolytic, colicin V positive, and serum resistant. SH48 and HU849 are recombinant strains prepared from J96 DNA. They express mannose-sensitive or Gal-Gal pili, respectively, and therefore collectively exhibit the binding repertoire of the parent strain. P678-54 is a nonpiliated K-12 recipient. The functional attributes of pili purified from these recombinants were also determined (Table IV). HU849 pili agglutinate human erythrocytes and latex particles adsorbed with Syn Gal-Gal. SH48 pili agglutinate pig erythrocytes and latex particles adsorbed with Syn Man-Man. Thus, the adherence properties of the parent strain and both recombinants are conferred by two pilus proteins that are functionally and genetically distinct.

Table IV. BALB/c Mouse Urinary Tract Infection Model

| | | | Colonization | | | | Renal Invasion |
|---|---|---|---|---|---|---|---|
| | | | Urine | | Rt. Kidney | | Rt. Kidney‡ |
| Strain | Pilus Operon(s) | Inoculum | No.+/Total | R.C.D.* | No.+/Total | R.C.D. | No.+/No.Assessed |
| J96 | MS§ & Gal-Gal‖ | $10^5$ | 4/7 | 3.2 | 5/7 | 2.3 | N.D.¶ |
| | | $10^6$ | 8/8 | 5.0 | 9/9 | 4.4 | 9/9 |
| | | $10^8$ | 5/5 | 4.8 | 5/5 | 4.3 | 5/5 |
| HU849 | Gal-Gal | $10^6$ | 8/9 | 4.2 | 10/10 | 3.6 | 0/10 |
| SH48 | MS | $10^6$ | 4/8 | 1.4 | 0/8 | 0 | 0/8 |
| | | $10^8$ | N.D. | N.D. | 0/7 | 0 | N.D. |
| | | $10^{10}$ | N.D. | N.D. | 5/7 | 1.1 | N.D. |
| | | $10^{12}$ | N.D. | N.D. | 6/6 | 3.5 | 0/3 |
| P678-54 | None | $10^6$ | 0/11 | 0 | 0/11 | 0 | 0/5 |
| | | $10^{12}$ | 0/5 | 0 | 0/5 | 0 | N.D. |

*R.C.D.- Relative colonization density is expressed as the mean of the particular strain colonizing the urine or kidney per total number of inoculated mice.

‡ Renal Invasion- assessed by light microscopy.

§ MS- Mannose sensitive agglutination.

‖ Gal-Gal - αD Gal (1 →4) βD Gal agglutination.

¶ N.D.- not done

Strain J96, HU849, P678-54, or SH48 was administered by intraurethral catheterization (31). The mice were sacrificed at 48 hours and urine and renal colonization was determined by culture and renal invasion by light microscopy (Table IV). At challenge doses of $10^6$ or $10^8$ colony-forming units, J96 colonized the urine and kidneys in all mice. Histologic evidence of renal invasion was found in each of the 14 autopsied mice. In contrast, HU849 did not invade, although it colonized the urine in eight of nine mice and the kidneys in 10 of 10 mice. At a challenge dose of $10^6$ colony-forming units, SH48 colonized the urine in four of eight mice but did not colonize or invade the kidneys. P678-54 was unable to colonize the Balb/c mouse urinary tract. These data may be interpreted as follows: (1) Gal-Gal but not mannose-sensitive pili mediate renal colonization. The binding capacity of mannose-sensitive pili for mannose-containing receptor compounds on renal epithelium (Table II) may be abolished _in vivo_ by the Tamm-Horsfall glycoprotein in urine. However, at higher inocula ($10^{10}$ to $10^{12}$ colony-forming units) the mannose-sensitive recombinant successfully colonized renal epithelia, indicating that this inhibition of adherence could be overcome (Table IV). These results may be exemplary of a general principle of mucosal pathogenesis: (1) colonization is a function of the relative molar concentration in situ, of cell-bound and free receptor compounds and the affinity of bacterial binding organelles for each; and (2) colonization and invasion are distinct pathogenic events mediated by separate microbial molecules. In addition, colonization appears to precede and to be a prerequisite for invasion. This formulation was evaluated by determining the efficacy of Gal-Gal and mannose-sensitive pili as vaccines for the prevention of pyelonephritis (31).

Mannose-sensitive and Gal-Gal were purified to homogeneity from recombinant strains SH48 and HU849 and their antigenic cross-reactivity was assessed by a two-step competitive enzyme-linked immunosorbent assay with antiserum samples to each pilus preparation. Less than 5 percent shared antigenicity was detected (23). Therefore, the protection conferred by a Gal-Gal or mannose-sensitive pilus vaccine could be attributed to the homologous immunogen. Fifty micrograms of purified Gal-Gal or mannose-sensitive pili or somatic O immunogen (prepared from heat-killed organisms from strains J96 and P678-54) or saline solution were emulsified in complete Freund's adjuvant and administered to 16-week Balb/c mice by subcutaneous and intramuscular injection. Two weeks later the mice were challenged with $10^6$ colony-forming units of strain J96 by intraurethral catheterization. The immunogenicity of the somatic O and the two pilus vaccines was assessed as the specific IgG response in serum and found to be approximately the same. However, immunization with saline solution, the somatic immunogens, or pure mannose-sensitive pili did not block colonization or invasion (Table V). In contrast, the Gal-Gal pilus vaccine prevented the colonization of urine and kidney in 80 percent of the recipients; renal invasion occurred in only one of 11 mice. These data confirm the critical role of Gal-Gal pili in the pathogenesis of pyelonephritis and indicate that vaccines that block colonization also prevent invasion.

Table V. Vaccine Efficacy for the Prevention of Urinary Tract Infection by *E. coli* Strain J96*

| | J96 Colonization§ | | | | | J96 Renal Invasion |
|---|---|---|---|---|---|---|
| Immunogen‡ | Urine No.+/Total | R.C.D. | Rt Kidney No.+/Total | Lt Kidney No.+/Total | R.C.D. | Rt Kidney‖ No.+/Total Autopsied |
| Buffer Control | 8/8 | 4.6 | 8/8 | 8/8 | 4.2 | 4/4 |
| Somatic O P678-54 | 4/4 | 4.8 | 4/4 | 4/4 | 4.0 | 4/4 |
| Somatic O J96 | 4/4 | 5.0 | 4/4 | 4/4 | 4.5 | 4/4 |
| SH48 Pili (MS pili) | 8/8 | 5.0 | 8/8 | 8/8 | 5.0 | 4/4 |
| HU849 Pili (Gal-Gal pili) | 4/22 | 0.6 | 3/22 | 2/22 | 0.3 | 1/11 |

* Challenge dose: $10^6$ CFU by urethral intra-vesicular catherization two weeks after immunization.

‡ Administered to 16 week BALB/c mice in complete Freund's adjuvant by subcutaneous and intra-muscular injections.

§ Assessed by culture two days after challenge dose; R.C.D.- relative colonization density is expressed as the mean of J96 colonizing the urine or the kidney per total number of inoculated mice or the total number of kidneys examined, respectively.

‖ Assessed by light microscopy.

## STRUCTURE-FUNCTION ANALYSIS OF ISOLATED PILI

The covalent structure of Gal-Gal mannose-sensitive pili was studied to determine the chemical basis for their receptor binding and antigenic properties. Pili were purified from recombinant strains HU849 and SH48 and their subunit molecular weights estimated by sodium dodecyl sulfate-polyacrylamide gel electrophoresis. Mannose-sensitive pili only entered the gel after acid depolymerization according to the method of McMichael and Ou (32) and migrated with an Mr of 19 Kd and 17 Kd; the Mr of Gal-Gal pili was 17.5 Kd. Their amino acid compositions were similar but not identical. A large proportion of nonpolar hydrophobic residues was noted. Both contain two cysteine residues in disulfide linkage per subunit. The N-terminal amino acid sequences were determined by automated Edman degradation through residue 46 (Table III). Although the genes encoding these sequences were cloned from separate positions of the same chromosome, the pilus proteins were found to exhibit homology and are highly homologous with the published N-terminal sequences of five mannose-sensitive and five Gal-Gal pili from other uropathogenic E. coli (33,34). When the cysteine residues are aligned, 13 of the first 46 positions (27%) are homologous (23). Eight of the conserved residues are between positions 9 and 22, a region that exhibits the pattern -Gly-$X_1$-Val-$X_2$-Phe-$X_3$-Gly-$X_4$-Val-Val-Asx-Ala-$X_5$-Cys-, where the intervening residues (X) tend to be charged or polar uncharged. C-terminal homology may also exist. The HU849 Gal-Gal pilus C-terminal amino acid sequence was determined by automated Edman degradation of a tryptic fragment (23) and aligned for maximal homology with the published C-terminal sequence of two mannose-sensitive pili (Types 1B and 1C) deduced from the amino acids released by carboxypeptidase Y hydrolysis (34). The Gal-Gal and mannose-sensitive sequences are -Phe-Asn-Leu-Thr-Tyr-Gln-COOH and -Thr-Phe-Asn-Val-Tyr-Gln-COOH, respectively. These structural features, their carbohydrate-binding properties, and the chromosomal location of both operons suggest that mannose-sensitive and Gal-Gal binding pili arose from a common ancestral gene and that the conserved regions are functionally or physically critical. Conversely, their functional differences suggest that relatively little homology exists in portions of these molecules which encompass the receptor binding domain. It must be presumed that the receptor specificities of mannose-sensitive and Gal-Gal pili confer a selective advantage in separate ecologic niches characterized by different host molecules in mucus or on cell surfaces. The discovery of chromosomally determined mannose-resistant pili of X specificity (24) from uropathogenic E. coli which agglutinate human erythrocytes in the presence of D-mannose and Syn Gal-Gal indicates that the binding repertoire of these organelles may be extensive.

## CLINICAL APPLICATIONS: RECURRENT INFECTIONS OF THE URINARY TRACT

A small proportion of women experience recurrent infections of the urinary tract. No anatomic or physiologic abnormality can be demonstrated in most. However, their vaginal or voided epithelial cells appear to bind larger numbers of uropathogenic E. coli than do cells from normal control subjects (4,17,35). Accordingly the urogenital mucosa of infection-prone women may exhibit a relatively greater density of cell surface Gal-Gal pilus receptor molecules. Recognizing that these compounds are glycolipids of the globoseries and also antigens of the P blood group system (21-23), Lonberg et al. (36) examined the relation between P blood group phenotype and the risk of recurrent pyelonephritis in girls. The P1 phenotype was more common among infection prone patients without vesicoureteral reflux than among normal children. Thus, the epithelial surfaces of the P1 phenotype may elaborate more pilus receptor molecules than those of the P2 phenotype (36). In summary, the density on urogenital mucosa of the Gal-Gal pilus receptor may be associated with the P1 blood group phenotype and these, in turn, correlate with infection risk. The validity of this proposal must now be assessed with quantitative determinations of pilus receptor density in appropriate tissues of infection-prone and normal women.

## CLINICAL APPLICATIONS: MOLECULAR STRATEGIES FOR THE PREVENTION OF PYELONEPHRITIS

The elucidation of microbial and host determinants of pathogenicity has led us to propose a two-phase strategy for the prevention of pyelonephritis. (1) "Receptor-dense" persons (the infection prone population) are identified by a quantitative assay of cell surface pilus receptor glycoconjugates. Anti-receptor antibody (vide supra) is employed with voided uroepithelial or vaginal cells to assess receptor content. (2) The infection-prone group is immunized with a vaccine composed of Gal-Gal pili. An alternative modality is derived from the observation that soluble receptor analogs may compete with cell surface receptor compounds for bacterial ligands and thereby block their binding capacity (29). Indeed, the oligosaccharide moiety of globoside, the P antigen of the P blood group system, effectively inhibited colonization of the Balb/c mouse urinary tract by a pyelonephritogenic E. coli strain (29). The prevention of pyelonephritis by soluble receptor analogs and vaccination is under active study in several centers. Clinical trials will determine their place in therapeutics relative to the proven efficacy of antimicrobial therapy.

## ACKNOWLEDGEMENT

We thank Irevis Josefina de Romero for skillful technical assistance and Milly Robinson for manuscript preparation.

## REFERENCES

1. Vosti, K.L., L.M. Goldberg, A.S. Monto and L.A. Rantz. Host-parasite interaction in patients with infections due to Escherichia coli. I. The serogrouping of E. coli from intestinal and extraintestinal sources, J. Clin. Invest. 43:2377 (1964).
2. Turck, M. and R.G. Petersdorf. The epidemiology of non-enteric Escherichia coli infections: prevalence of serological groups, J. Clin. Invest. 41:1760 (1962).
3. Svanborg-Eden, C. Attachment of Escherichia coli to human urinary tract epithelial cells, Scand. J. Infect. Dis. 15(suppl): 1 (1978).
4. Fowler, J.E. and T.A. Stamey. Studies of introital colonization in women with recurrent urinary infections. VII. The role of bacterial adherence, J. Urol. 117:472 (1977).
5. Hagberg, L., U. Jodal, T. Korhonen, G. Lidin-Janson, U. Lindberg and C. Svanborg-Eden. Adhesion, hemagglutination and virulence of Escherichia coli causing urinary tract infections, Infect. Immun. 31:564 (1981).
6. Binns, M., D. Davies and K. Hardy. Cloned fragments of the plasmid Col V, I-K94 specifying virulence and serum resistance, Nature 279:778 (1979).
7. Bjorksten, B. and B. Kaijser. Interaction of human serum and neutrophils with Escherichia coli strains: differences between strains isolated from urine of patients with pyelonephritis or asymptomatic bacteriuria, Infect. Immun. 22:308 (1978).
8. Olling, S. Sensitivity of gram negative bacilli to the serum bactericidal activity: a marker of host-parasite relationship in acute and persisting infections, Scand. J. Infect. Dis. 10(suppl): 1 (1977).
9. Minshew, B.H., J. Jorgensen, G. Counts and S. Falkow. Association

of hemolysin production, hemagglutination of human erythrocytes, and virulence for chicken embryos of extraintestinal Escherichia coli isolates, Infect. Immun. 20:50 (1977).
10. Cooke, M. and S. Ewins. Properties of strains of Escherichia coli isolated from a variety of sources, J. Med. Microbiol. 8:107 (1975).
11. Evans, D., D. Evans, C. Hohne, M.A. Noble, E.V. Haldane, H. Lior and L.S. Young. Hemolysin and K antigens in relation to serotype and hemagglutination type of Escherichia coli isolated from extraintestinal infections, J. Clin. Microbiol. 13:171 (1981).
12. Brooks, H., F. O'Grady, M. McSherry and W. Cattel. Uropathogenic properties of Escherichia coli in recurrent urinary-tract infection, J. Med. Microbiol. 13:57 (1980).
13. Davies, D., F. Falkiner and K. Hardy. Colicin V production by clinical isolates of Escherichia coli, Infect. Immun. 31:574 (1981).
14. Minshew, B.H., J. Jorgensen, M. Swanstrum, G. Grootes-Reuvecamp and S. Falkow. Some characteristics of Escherichia coli strains isolated from extraintestinal infections of humans, J. Infect. Dis. 137:648 (1978).
15. Svanborg-Eden, C., B. Eriksson and L. Hanson. Adhesion of Escherichia coli to human uroepithelial cells in vitro, Infect. Immun. 18:767 (1977).
16. Leffler, H., H. Lomberg, E. Gotschlich, et al. Chemical and clinical studies on the interaction of Escherichia coli with host glycolipid receptors in urinary tract infection, Scand. J. Infect. Dis. 33(suppl):46 (1981).
17. Kallenius, G. and J. Winberg. Bacterial adherence to periurethral epithelial cells in girls prone to urinary tract infections, Lancet II:240 (1978).
18. Orskov, I., A. Ferencz, F. Orskov. Tamm-Horsfall protein or uromucoid is the normal urinary slime that traps Type 1 fimbriated Escherichia coli, Lancet 1:887 (1980).
19. Salit, I. and E. Gotschlich. Hemagglutination by purified type 1 Escherichia coli pili, J. Exp. Med. 146:1169 (1977).
20. Salit, I. and E. Gorschlich. Type 1 Escherichia coli pili: characterization of binding to monkey kidney cells, J. Exp. Med. 146:1182 (1977).
21. Leffler, H. and C. Svanborg-Eden. Chemical identification of a glycosphingolipid receptor for Escherichia coli attaching to human urinary tract epithelial cells agglutinating human erythrocytes, FEMS Microbiol. Lett. 8:127 (1980).
22. Kallenius, G., R. Mollby, S.B. Svenson, J. Winberg, A. Lundblad, S. Svensson and B. Cedergren. The $p^k$ antigen as receptor for the hemagglutination of pyelonephritogenic Escherichia coli, FEMS Microbiol. Lett. 7:297 (1980).
23. O'Hanley, P., D. Lark, S. Normark, S. Falkow and G. Schoolnik. Mannose-sensitive and Gal-Gal binding Escherichia coli pili from recombinant strains, J. Exp. Med. 158:1713 (1983).
24. Vaisanen, V., J. Elo, L. Tallgren, H. Shtonen, P. Helena Makela, C. Svanborg-Eden, G. Kallenius, S.B. Svenson, H. Hultberg and T. Korhonen. Mannose-resistant hemagglutination and P antigen recognition characteristic of E. coli causing primary pyelonephritis, Lancet II:1366 (1981).
25. Sheladia, W., J. Chambers, J. Guevara and D. Evans. Isolation purification and partial characterization of type V-A hemagglutinin from Escherichia coli GV-12, O1:H, J. Bacteriol. 152:757 (1982).
26. Kallenius, G., R. Mollby, S. Svenson, I. Helin, H. Hultberg, B. Cedegren and J. Winberg. Occurence of P-fimbriated Escherichia coli in urinary tract infections, Lancet II:1369 (1981).
27. Hull, R., R. Gill, P. Hsu, B. Minshew and S. Falkow. Construction and expression of recombinant plasmids encoding Type 1 or D-mannose-resistant pili from a urinary tract infection Escherichia

coli isolate; Infect. Immun. 33:933 (1981).
28. Kaijser, B. and P. Larsson. Experimental acute pyelonephritis caused by enterobacteria in animals. A review, J. Urol. 127:786 (1982).
29. Svanborg-Eden, C., R. Freter, L. Hagberg, et al. Inhibition of experimental ascending urinary tract infection by an epithelial cell-surface receptor analogue, Nature 298:560 (1982).
30. Tamm, I. and F. Horsfall. A mucoprotein derived from human urine which reacts with influenza, mumps, and Newcastle disease viruses, J. Exp. Med. 95:71 (1952).
31. O'Hanley, P., D. Lark, S. Falkow and G. Schoolnik. Molecular basis of Escherichia coli colonization of the upper urinary tract in Balb/c mice: Gal-Gal pili immunization prevents E. coli pyelonephritis in the Balb/c mouse model of human pyelonephritis, J. Clin. Invest. 75:347 (1985).
32. McMichael, J. and J. Ou. Structure of common pili from Escherichia coli, J. Bacteriol. 138:969 (1979).
33. Svanborg-Eden, C., E. Gotschlich, T. Korhonen, H. Leffler and G. Schoolnik. Aspects on structure and function of pili on uropathogenic Escherichia coli; Prog. Allergy 33:189 (1983).
34. Klemm, P., I. Orskov and F. Orskov. F7 and type 1-like fimbriae from three Escherichia coli strains isolated from urinary tract infections: protein chemical and immunological aspects, Infect. Immun. 36:462 (1982).
35. Svanborg-Eden, C. and U. Jodal. Attachment of Escherichia coli to sedimented epithelial cells from urinary tract infection-prone and healthy children, Infect. Immun. 26:837 (1979).
36. Lomberg, H., L. Hanson, B. Jacobsson, U. Jodal, H. Leffler and C. Svanborg-Eden. Correlation of P blood group, vesicoureteral reflux, and bacterial attachment in patients with recurrent pyelonephritis, N. Engl. J. Med. 308:1189 (1983).

ACKNOWLEDGEMENT

This work was supported by a grant from the Cetus Corporation and Public Health Grant A1-18719 from the National Institutes of Health, Bethesda, MD. Dr. Schoolnik is a Fellow of the John A. Hartford Foundation. Dr. Lark is a Fellow of the American Urological Association. Requests for reprints should be addressed to Dr. Gary Schoolnik, Department of Medicine, Division of Infectious Diseases, Stanford University Medical School, Stanford, California 94305.

# BACTERIURIA SCREENING:

# EVALUATION OF CURRENT METHODS

Alan T. Evangelista

Microbiology Department
Cooper Hospital/University Medical Center
Camden, New Jersey 08103

## INTRODUCTION

Diagnostic screens for patient specimens of high frequency such as blood and urine are advantageous in the current health care climate which places emphasis on cost containment and the rapid turnaround time of result reporting. Over the past few years rapid diagnostic methods for the detection of bacteriuria have increased in availability for the clinical microbiology laboratory. The advantages and limitations of these new systems can be evaluated through the performance of carefully designed comparative studies with reference urine culture methods. By reviewing published reports as well as conducting in-house parallel studies microbiologists can evaluate the newer methods in terms of sensitivity, specificity and predictive values. Additional parameters to be considered during an evaluation include workload efficiency based on time studies, impact on routine workflow, hands-on technologist time, total turnaround time and cost effectiveness. Historically, microbiologists and other lab professionals have approached new technology either directly or indirectly with these parameters in mind. However, under the new hospital Medicare prospective payment programs based on diagnostic related groups (DRG) this approach to new methodologies is now essential in the day-to-day operation of the lab.

The bacteriuria screens that are currently available can be classified into manual, semi-automated and automated systems. Manual methods include staining/ microscopy as well as chemical and enzyme-based screens. The semi-automated systems utilize filtration/ colorimetry and the technology of bioluminescence. The automated systems are growth dependent screens using light scatter and photometry as their method of detection. Before evaluating the efficacy and limitations of each method the purpose of urine screening should be clearly stated. A hospital microbiology laboratory that processes 20-50 urine specimens per day requires a urine screening method that can rapidly eliminate negative specimens, thereby directing efforts to the identification and susceptibility testing of positive specimens. In contrast a low volume laboratory or physicians office that handles only a few outpatient specimens per day may need just a quick yes or no answer for a community-acquired urinary tract infection (UTI) and may find it clinically acceptable and cost effective to wait 24-48 hours for a more definitive answer.

## CLINICAL-UTI SYNDROMES

The current bacteriuria screens have detection thresholds of either $10^4$ colony forming units (cfu) of bacteria per ml of urine or $10^5$ cfu/ml. Since the term urinary tract infection applies to several distinct clinical syndromes it is essential to consider each one separately in terms of screening for bacteriuria and pyuria (Table 1). Acute pyelonephritis, a symptomatic upper UTI involving kidneys and often causing systemic symptoms, has been associated with a bacterial threshold of $\geq 10^5$ cfu/ml of urine in 96% of patients (1). This threshold provides optimal separation of infection from contamination of clean-voided urine and is well-suited for bacteriuria screens. Pyuria as defined by >10 white blood cells per $mm^3$ is almost always present and a screen for pyuria could be an aid in the diagnosis of pyelonephritis. A second UTI syndrome defined as asymptomatic bacteriuria is found predominantly in women and in patients with long-term indwelling catheters. The quantitative definition of asymptomatic bacteriuria has been set at a bacterial threshold of $10^5$ cfu/ml of urine (2). The prevalence of this condition in women increases with age from 2% at 10 years of age to 6% at 60 years of age (3). The prevalence during pregnancy is approximately 5% with 73% of women with bacteriuria having $> 10^5$ cfu/ml of urine (4). This second UTI syndrome is also seen with very high prevalence (nearly 100% ) in patients who have indwelling catheters on a long-term basis (5). Thus, despite the varying degress of prevalence of bacteriuria in these different asymptomatic patient populations a bacteriuria screen would be useful in identifying those urine specimens with $\geq 10^5$ cfu/ml. However, a pyuria screen would not be as useful since only 50% of urine specimens have been shown to be positive for pyuria in asymptomatic UTI (2).

Table 1. Clinical urinary tract infection syndromes and usefulness of bacteriuria and pyuria screening

| UTI Syndrome | | threshold cfu/ml | pyuria > 10 WBC/$mm^3$ | bacteriuria screen efficacy |
|---|---|---|---|---|
| I. | acute pyelonephritis | $\geq 10^5$ | >98% | + |
| II. | asymptomatic bacteriuria | $\geq 10^5$ | 50% | + |
| III. | catheter-associated inf. | $\geq 10^4$ | 70% | +/- |
| IV. | acute dysuria & frequ. | $\geq 10^2$ | 90% | - |

Catheter-associated urinary tract infection represents a third UTI syndrome (Table 1). Approximately 10-20 percent of patients with short-term cathether courses (<1 week) have demonstrated bacterial infections in bladder urine of $> 10^5$ cfu/ml (6,7). However, a bacterial threshold of $\geq 10^4$ cfu/ml may be the most appropriate for catheter-associated infection since individuals with urine specimens of $10^4$ cfu/ml are likely to progress to $> 10^5$/ml with the same organism on the following day (8). Therefore, for short term catheterized patients the usefulness of a bacteriuria screen would be limited to those systems capable of detecting $10^4$ cfu/ml with acceptable sensitivity. Since many catheter-associated infections are also asymptomatic, a pyuria screen would be of limited value. The fourth UTI syndrome has been referred to as the acute urethral syndrome (9) or the acute dysuria and urinary frequency syndrome (8). This symptomatic lower UTI is one of the most common illnesses of young women with a peak prevalence rate of 9% in the 15-24 year old range and gradually dropping to 4% at age 60 (3,10). Since only 50% of cases have a bacterial threshold of > $10^5$ cfu/ml, the more recent recommendations have been to use the criterion of $\geq 10^2$ cfu/ml for the best separation of infected from uninfected women (9). This criterion, however, was based on a study population with a 52% prevalence rate of bacteriuria as determined by catheterization or suprapubic aspiration. With a high prevalence rate the threshold of $\geq 10^2$ cfu/ml yielded a 95% sensitivity and 85% specificity for identifying a UTI. Considering the difficulty in collecting an uncontaminated clean-voided urine sample from this population the $\geq 10^2$ cfu/ml threshold would produce a high number of false positives in most settings. Furthermore, neither bacteriuria screens nor the standard calibrated loop method can detect as low as $10^2$ cfu/ml and a more time-consuming tube dilution pour plate or spread plate method would be required. Therefore, a practical approach to the diagnosis of symptomatic lower UTI would be to perform a bacteriuria screen or culture with a $10^4$ cfu/ml threshold to identify 50-60% of the patients with this syndrome and to rely on a test for pyuria to identify patients who are abacteriuric by present screening methods. Over 90% of patients with acute dysuria and frequency syndrome are positive for pyuria and the combination of lower urinary tract symptoms and pyuria diagnostically suggests a treatable condition (11).

The laboratory performing the diagnostic evaluation of a urine specimen should be provided with certain patient and specimen demographics such as: patient's name, age, sex, admitting or current diagnosis, clinic or hospital location, date/time of collection and specimen type i.e. clean-voided or catheterized. With this information the specimen can be associated with one of the four UTI syndromes and handled accordingly. The decision to use a bacteriuria screen would be based on the type of specimen received, the specific patient population identified, and the previous organism occurrence rates for that population. The prevalence of certain organisms in a key factor since some bacteriuria screens may be poor at detecting gram positive cocci such as enterococci, Staph. saprophyticus and Group B streptococci. Some screens may also have difficulty in detecting yeasts and encapsulated gram negative rods.

## REFERENCE METHOD

A bacteriuria screen is evaluated by performing parallel testing with a reference urine culture method. The most frequently used method to enumerate bacteria is the calibrated loop procedure of semiquantitative colony counting on sheep blood agar. The more accurate tube dilution pour plate procedure is time-consuming and not a practical culture method for a busy clinical laboratory. Prior to an evaluation of a urine screen, the limitations of the calibrated loop technique should be addressed.

The volume of specimen delivered by a calibrated loop contributes the greatest variability to this method. Reproducibility in volume delivered has been reported at ±50% (12). The angle of sampling may also contribute to volume errors with the optimum angle being 45° (12). Hence the loop method must be recognized as only semiquantitative for purposes of parallel testing and for result reporting. The two standard loop sizes are .001 ml and .01 ml. The choice of loop size is based upon which threshold is to be used for a positive specimen, i.e. $10^4$ cfu/ml or $10^5$ cfu/ml of bacteria in urine. A reproducible colony count on an agar plate is 100 colonies with the loop method. Therefore, 100 colonies on a plate inoculated with .001 ml loop would represent $10^5$ cfu/ml and on a plate inoculated with a .01 ml loop would represent $10^4$ cfu/ml. Overall, the .001 ml calibrated loop is only accurate at bacterial counts of $10^5$ cfu ml and $\geq 10^6$ cfu/ml and the .01 ml calibrate loop is accurate at counts of $10^4$ cfu/ml and $\geq 10^5$ cfu/ml. Thus, parallel studies that evaluate the accuracy of a bacteriuria screen at $10^4$ cfu/ml should use a .01 ml loop to most accurately determine colony counts for that threshold.

## MANUAL METHODS

The oldest and most traditional method of urine screening is the Gram stain. The presence of greater than one organism per oil immersion field from uncentrifuged urine has been reported to correlate with a colony count of $\geq 10^5$ cfu/ml (2). In a recent study of 1055 urine specimens, as shown in Table 2, the Gram stain urine screen had a reported sensitivity of 84% and a specificty of 95% (13). The positive and negative predictive values were 80% and 97% respectively. Since the prevalence of UTI in the general population is relatively low at 25-30%, the negative predictive values for most urine screens are typically very high at 95-98% (Table 2). However, a more important criterion to focus on is the sensitivity of the test i.e. the % of people with UTI who are detected by the screen. A sensitivity of 84% for the Gram stain translates into a false negative rate of 16% which means that 16% of patients with actual UTI's will be missed by this screen. Advantages of the Gram stain are the low cost of $.30-.45/test, relative ease of performance, and the ability to identify organism morphology which aids in selecting appropriate antimicrobial therapy. Disadvantages of this urine screen are the low sensitivity compared to other manual methods and the fact that it is a manual method requiring microscopy time with the added eye strain of viewing several oil immersion fields. There is often little difference between a positive and negative result with positives often having as few as 1 organism/ field. This method is better suited for an occasional specimen rather than the screening of large numbers of specimens.

Table 2. Comparison of manual methods

| | Gram[a] Stain | Acridine[a] Orange | LN[b] Strip | Dipslide[c] |
|---|---|---|---|---|
| specimens | 1055 | 1055 | 2782 | 500 |
| threshold (cfu/ml) | $10^5$ | $10^5$ | $10^5$ | $10^4$ |
| sensitivity % | 84 | 92 | 87 | 93 |
| specificity% | 95 | 65 | 67 | 100 |
| pred value pos % | 80 | 36 | 29 | 100 |
| pred value neg % | 97 | 97 | 97 | 98 |
| UTI's missed % | 16 | 8 | 13 | 7 |
| pigmenters % | - | - | 2 | - |

a - Crout and Tilton (13). b - Bartlett (14). c - Granato (15).

The second microscopic method in Table 2 for the detection of bacteriuria is the fluorescent acridine orange stain. This method is easier to read than the Gram stain because a fluorescent microscope with high dry magnification (400 x) is used for screening. Greater than 5 organisms per high power field from unspun urine correlates with $\geq 10^5$ cfu/ml and the sensitivity of the acridine orange stain is slightly higher at 92% when compared with the Gram stain (13). However, nonspecific fluorescence results in more false positives and the specificity has been reported to be only 65% (13). The number of patients with UTI's that are missed by the acridine orange stain is 8%. As with any microscopy procedure, the acridine orange stain is time-consuming when screening large numbers of urine specimens. Compared to the Gram stain, however, the acridine orange stain requires about a third less time to perform and is about half the cost at $.20/test.

A biochemical method for detecting bacteriuria has been developed in the configuration of a urine dipstick, the Chemistrip LN (Biodynamics/ Boehringer Mannheim). The LN strip contains two reagent patches for the detection of leukocyte esterase and nitrite repectively. A positive test for leukocyte esterase can be an indicator of a significant pyuria and a positive urine nitrite test should correlate with those urinary tract infections that are caused by organisms capable of reducing nitrate to nitrite. When either one or both tests are positive the sensitivity has been reported to be 87% at a threshold of $10^5$ cfu/ml (14). An advantage of the Chemstrip LN is that it is truly a rapid test. The leukocyte esterase is read a 1 minute and verified at 2 minutes and the nitrite is read at 30 seconds. The strip is also inexpensive at $.25/test which is comparable to the cost of staining methods. However, as showin in Table 2, the LN strip demonstrated a low specificity of 67% due specifically to a substantial number of false positive leukocyte esterase tests (14). While the predictive value of a negative test was high at 97% the number of UTI's missed was 17% (Table 2), a more significant limitation for a procedure designed to screen out negative urine specimens. Additional limitations which could contribute to false negative leukocyte esterase tests are high levels of albumin ($\geq$ 500 mg/dl) in the urine, and the presence of cephalexin and gentamicin. False positive esterase could result from a voided urine not collected cleanly containing leukocytes from a source external to the renal urinary tract. However, some false positives may be misclassified due to the patient population having $< 10^5$ cfu/ml in the reference culture method. These patients may belong to the acute dysuria female outpatient population where the definition of UTI would be primarily pyuria with very low bacterial count. The nitrite test can result in a false negative following ingestion of large amounts of ascorbic acid from vitamins and fruit juices. The test may also be negative if the UTI is caused by organisms that do not reduce nitrate such as enterococci and most yeasts. To optimize the nitrite reaction, the patient's diet should include vegetables, an important cource of nitrates and the urine should be allowed to sit in the bladder for at least 4 hours, hence the importance of a first morning specimen. Even though the Chemstrip LN has several limitations, one of its primary attributes is the detection of pyuria in the carefully defined female outpatient population with the acute dysuria and frequency syndrome.

The fourth manual method presented in Table 2 is a bacteriuria screen requiring overnight incubation, the dipslide culture system. An evaluation of the Uricult (Orion Diagnostics) resulted in a 93% sensitivity and 100% specificity for a $10^4$ cfu/ml threshold when compared to the calibrated loop method (15). In this study the 2 x 5 cm. plastic paddle was coated on both sides with selective agar media: MacConkey agar for gram negatives and CLED agar (cystine-lactose-electrolyte deficient) for gram positives and yeast. Since no false positives were detected in the study the specificity was 100%. An advantage of this method is the simplicity of use of dipping the paddle into a well-mixed urine specimen or pouring the specimen over the surface of the paddle. The system also allows direct on-site inoculation of urine eliminating transport problems with the associated potential for bacterial overgrowth of the specimen. However, the CLED agar does not support the growth of alpha and beta hemolytic streptococci and Corynebacterium sp. which can be causative agents of UTI. Furthermore, the dipslide method is not a rapid screen. After overnight incubation enumeration of bacteria on a small paddle surface is more difficult to interpret than on an agar plate. Paddle colony density is compared to a model chart and accurately differentiating between $10^4$ cfu/ml, $10^5$ cfu/ml and > $10^5$ cfu/ml may pose problems if colonies are not evenly distributed. Moreover, to select isolated colonies for identification and susceptibility testing may require a subculture, delaying result reporting by an additional 24 hr. The dipslide method seems to be better suited for a private physicians office than for diagnostic microbiology laboratory. At a cost of \$.80 - \$1.00 for any one of the 22 commercial sources of dipslides and agar trays a diagnostic lab could more cost effectively perform the calibrated loop method. However, physician in a private office seeking a yes or no answer to a community acquired UTI in 24 hours may find the dipslide very useful, especially when the patient would be treated empirically for the UTI and subculture with susceptibility testing would not be deemed necessary.

SEMI-AUTOMATED METHODS

The most rapid bacteriuria screen using an instrument is the Bac-T-Screen (Vitek Systems, formerly sold by Marion Scientific). The urine screen is performed in 2 minutes in which the specimen is passed through a filter paper disk attached to a card, and then stained with safranin O dye and rinsed with decolorizer. The pink color intensity on the filter is read by a colorimeter and is proportional to the cfu/ml of bacteria in urine. The Bac-T-Screen (BTS) can detect bacteria at a threshold of $10^4$ cfu/ml with reported sensitivities of 88-89% (16,17). Therefore, UTI's missed by this instrument are in the range of 11-12% of patients (Table 3). The sensitivity of the instrument has been reported as high as 98% when a positive threshold of $10^5$ cfu/ml was used (18). Not all urine specimens can be porcessed by this method. Some urines leave a residual pigment on the filter which gives an uninterpretable result while other specimens contain WBC's and/or mucous and do not pass through the filter and are termed cloggers. The comparative studies listed in Table 3 recorded substantial numbers of pigmenters and cloggers represented by 16-17% of urine specimens. Another limitation of the Bac-T-Screen is the large number of false positives reported as low specificities of 65-66% (16, 17). This would necessitate the culturing of many negative urine specimens initially screened as positive by the Bac-T-Screen.

Table 3. Comparison of semi-automated methods

| | BTS[a] | BTS[b] | Lumac[c] | Lumac[d] |
|---|---|---|---|---|
| specimens | 246 | 426 | 2000 | 600 |
| threshold (cfu/ml) | $10^4$ | $40^4$ | $50^4$ | $10^4$ |
| sensitivity % | 88 | 89 | 96.4 | 99 |
| specificity% | 66 | 65 | 71 | 80 |
| pred value pos % | 43 | 49 | 40 | 61 |
| pred value neg % | 94.2 | 94 | 99 | 99.7 |
| UTI's missed % | 12 | 11 | 3.6 | 1 |
| cloggers/pigmenters % | 16 | 17 | - | - |

a - Cantrill and Stokes (16)
b - Hoyt and Ellner (17)
c - Park et al (19)
d - Evangelista and DeObaldia (20)

The second semi-automated method compared in Table 3 uses the principle of bioluminescence to detect bacteriuria. The systems available commercially are Lumac (3M Company) and Monolight (Analytical Luminescence Laboratory) with detection times of 35 minutes and 15 minutes respectively. Bacteria are enumerated by first releasing adenosine triphosphate (ATP) from the bacteria in the urine sample, and then quantitating the ATP by the firefly luciferin/luciferase bioluminescent reaction. One quantum of light is emmitted for each molecule of luciferin oxidized which consumes one molecule of ATP. The reaction occurs in a photometer and the relative lightunits (RLU) detected at 560 nm wavelength are directly proportional to the cfu/ml of bacteria in urine. The Lumac system has reported sensitivities of 96.4% and 99% at a threshold of $10^4$ cfu/ml (19,20). This system is a highly sensitive method for detecting bacteria in urine. Unfortunately, like the Bac-T-Screen, the Lumac suffers from a high degree of false positives with specificities of only 71% and 80% (12,20). However, negative urine specimens are identified by the bioluminescent method with a high degree of confidence since only 1-3.6% of patients with UTI's are missed (Table 3) and negative predictive values have been reported at 99% and 99.7% (19,20). The individual cost per test ranges from $1.00 to $1.25 which is comparable to the Bac-T-Screen. While the individual costs are reasonable, the semi-automated methods can be costly to perform due to the large numbers of false positives which are both screened and cultured. Instrument down time and quality control set-up time for colorimetry and bioluminescent photometry must also be considered with respect to laboratory workflow.

AUTOMATED METHODS

Three automated systems are presently available for bacteriuria screening and all three systems detect bacterial growth over time using photometric analysis: Autobac MTS (Organon Teknika, formerly sold by General Diagnostics), Vitek AMS (Vitek Systems) and the Abbott MS-2/Avantage (Abbott Laboratories). In the Autobac system bacterial growth is monitered by changes in light scatter in a multichambered optical cuvette. In one study 66% of posiive urines were detected within 2 hours and 95% of urines were detected at a threshold of $10^5$ cfu/ml at 5 hours (21). The Abbott MS-2 monitors bacterial growth in a single ampvette at 5 minute intervals by a series of light-emitting diodes (LED's). A positive urine result is printed when an increase in turbidity is first detected, and specimens are monitored up to a maximum incubation time of 5 hours. The Vitek AMS differes from the other two automated systems by enumerating and identifying the nine organisms most often associated with UTI's. A sealed plastic card containing 30 wells of dehydrated selective media and divided into 3 sections is inoculated with three urine specimens. The inoculated cards are placed in a reader-incubator and read hourly by LED's for turbidometric changes. Results of most positive urines are printed out within 4 to 9 hours and the cards are read up to a maximum of 13 hours.

A comparison of all three automated systems is shown in Table 4 and the sensitivities for the detection of probable pathogens in urine were all 96% for the Autobac, Vitek AMS and MS-2/ Avantage (22). Only 4% of patients with significant UTI's at the $10^5$ cfu/ml threshold were missed by these three systems (Table 4). The average detection time for a positive specimen with $10^5$ cfu/ml of bacteria in urine was 1.9 hours for the MS-2, 2.3 hours for Autobac and 5.0 hours for the AMS (22).

Table 4. Comparison of automated methods

| | Automac[a] MTS | Vitek[a] AMS | Abbott[a] MS-2 |
|---|---|---|---|
| specimens | 1200 | 1200 | 1200 |
| breakpoint (cfu/ml) | $10^5$ | $10^5$ | $10^5$ |
| sensitivity % b | 96 | 96 | 96 |
| specificity% | 84 | 72 | 87 |
| pred value pos % | 63 | 49 | 65 |
| pred value neg % | 95 | 93 | 92 |
| UTI's missed% | 4 | 4 | 4 |

a - Pezzlo, et al. (22)
b - probable pathogens

JUSTIFICATION

The justification of any rapid system is usually thought of in terms of patient care and laboratory/hospital economics. The bacteriuria screens certainly have the ability to provide an earlier diagnostic result when compared to conventional urine culture. Faster turnaround time translates into an earlier clinical decision for the physician and perhaps a decreased length of stay for an inpatient. Moreover, a rapid negative answer would impact the pharmacy and hospital budget through the avoidance of unnecessary antimicrobial therapy. Theoretically, the laboratory would save money from an efficient and accurate negative urine screen by eliminating culture costs for 70-80% of urine specimens. However, in practical terms for the laboratory budget, a urine screen costs more to perform. The cost of a urine culture by calibrated loop method using three plates is approximately $.80 and using the bioluminescent screen as an example, the screen cost is $1.10. With a workload of 30 urines/day the lab materials cost for initial processing by standard plate method would be $24.00/day (30 x $.80). The use of a urine screen with 20% false positives could result in 18 urines screened as negative for only $19.80/day (18 x $1.10) but with the combined cost of a screen plus culture the 12 urines screened as positive would cost $22.80/day (12 x $1.90). Therefore, a laboratory using a urine screen would spend a total of $42.60/day or an excess of $18.60/day over culture alone. The justification for the cost of a urine screen could not be based on the laboratory budget alone but would have to include the potential impact on the pharmacy budget. The cost to the hospital of empiric UTI therapy with ampicillin P.O. 500 mg q 6h is $7.00 /day, with trimethoprim sulfamethoxazole P.O. 160/800 mg q 12h is $4.00/day, and with tobramycin IV 1.6 mg/kg q 8h is $35.00/day. Thus, the avoidance of using empiric therapy in just a few patients would make up for the extra laboratory costs

In addition to financial considerations, the overall evaluation of a urine screen should include the impact of the screen on laboratory workload and workflow. In our hands the time required to inoculate a urine by the calibrated loop method and read a negative culture result was 4.3 minutes/ specimen. In contrast, processing a negative urine with the Lumac screen including instrument QC per batch of 10 specimens required only 2.9 minutes/ specimen. However, since all screen positives were both screened and cultured the use of a urine screen required an average of 0.3 minutes more per specimen than manually plating all specimens. The implementation of a urine screen would usually require a new workstation in addition to more hands-on time as an impact on the microbiology laboratory. The trade-off is improved turnaround time for 60% of urine specimens. Instrument failure and reagent not performing within the quality control values are aspects of an evaluation that can only be appreciated by performing an in-house parallel study. Certainly, additional modifications and improvements to all of the semi-automated and automated systems would be welcomed by the evaluators and users of these instruments.

## CONCLUSION

In reviewing the current bacteriuria screens that are available today, none have the ability to completely duplicate the accuracy of the standard calibrated loop method. A major advantage of urine screens is the improved turnaround time for a negative result. However, it is essential to appreciate the limitations of each method including the calibrated loop. Furthermore the use of a bacteriuria screen is dependent on the association of a urine specimen with a clinical UTI syndrome identified by the lab requisition slip. Since bacteriuria screens perform better at a $10^5$ cfu/ml threshold than at $10^4$ cfu/ml they may not be applicable to catheterized specimens and the addition of a pyuria screen may be helpful in the clearly defined female outpatient with symptomatic lower UTI. Finally, the value of any urine screen or culture in establishing the diagnosis of a UTI is primarily dependent on the proper collection and delivery of the urine specimen itself.

## REFERENCES


1. Kass, E.H. Bacteriuria and the diagnosis of infections of the urinary tract. Arch. Intern. Med. 100: 709-714, 1957.
2. Kass, E.H., and M. Finland. Asymptomatic infections of the urinary tract. Trans. Assoc. Am. Physicians 69: 56-63, 1956.
3. Sabath, L.D. and D. Charles. Urinary tract infections in the female. Obstet. Gynecol. 55: 1625-1705, 1980.
4. McFadyen, I.R. S.J. Eykyn, M.H.N. Gardner, et al. Bacteriuria in pregnancy. J. Obstet. Gynaecol. 80: 385-405, 1973.
5. Warren, J.W., J.H. Tenney, J.M. Hoopes, H.L. Muncie and W.C. Anthony. A prospective microbiologic study of bacteriuria in patients with chronic indwelling catheters. J. Infect. Dis. 146: 719-723, 1982.
6. Platt, R., B.F. Polk, B. Murdock and B. Rosner. Mortality associated withnosocomial urinary tract infection. N. Engl. J. Med. 307: 637-642, 1982.
7. Garibaldi, R.A., J.P. Burke, M.L. Dickman, and C.B. Smith. Factors predisposing to bacteriuria during indwelling urethral catheterization. N. Engl. J. Med. 291: 215-219, 1974.
8. Platt, R. Quantitative definition of bacteriuria. Am. J. Med 75 1B: 44-52, 1983.
9. Stamm, W.E., K.F. Wagner, R. Amsel et al. Courses of the acute urethral syndrome. N. Engl. J. Med. 303: 409-415, 1980.
10. Mond, N.C., A. Percival, J.D. Williams and W. Brumfitt. Presentation, diagnosis and treatment of urinary tract infections in general practice. Lancet 1: 514-516, 1965.
11. Stamm, W.E. Interpretation of urine cultures. Clin. Micobiol. Newsl. 5: 15-17, 1983.
12. Albers, A.C. and R.D. Fletcher. Accuracy of the calibrated loop transfer. J. Clin. Microbiol. 18: 40-42, 1983.

13. Crout, F.V. and R.C. Tilton. Rapid screening of urine by gram stain, acridine orange stain, and Autobac MTS. Abstr. Annu. Meet. Am. Soc. Microbiol. C2: 312, 1983.
14. Bartlett, R.C., D.O'Neill and J.C. McLaughlin. Detection of bacteriuria by leukocyte esterase, nitrite, and the Automicrobic System. Am. J. Clin. Pathol. 82: 683-687, 1984.
15. Granato, P.A. Evaluation of a dip-slide device for enumeration of bacteria in urine. Lab. Med. 11: 246-250, 1980.
16. Cantrill, H.F. and B.H. Stokes. Comparison of Bac-T-Screen, leukocyte esterase and nitrite strips to conventional urine cultures. Abstr. Annu. Meet. Interscience Conf. Antimicrob. Agents Chemother. 733: 219, 1983.
17. Hoyt, S.M. and P.D. Ellner. Evaluation of the bacteriuria detection device. J. Clin. Microbiol. 18:882-884,1983.
18. David, J.R., C.E. Stager and G.F. Araj. Clinical laboratory evaluation of a bacteriuria detection device for urine screening. Am. J. Clin. Pathol. 81: 48-53, 1984.
19. Park, C.H., D.L. Hixon, C.C. McClintock et al. Rapid detection of insignificant bacteriuria by concomitant use of Lumac System and Gram's stain. Am. J. Clin. Pathol. 82: 593-596, 1984.
20. Evangelista, A.T. and J. DeObaldia. Bacteriuria screening by bioluminescence: clinical evaluation of the Lumac/3M system. Abstr. Annu. Meet. Am. Soc. Microbiol. C179: 266, 1984.
21. Kelly, M.T. and L.C. Balfour. Evaluation and optimization of urine screening by Autobac. J. Clin. Microbiol. 13: 677-680, 1981.
22. Pezzlo, M.T., G.L. Tan, E.M. Peterson and L.M. de la Maza. Screening of urine cultures by three automated systems. J. Clin. Microbiol 15: 468-474, 1982.

## LABORATORY ASPECTS OF CHLAMYDIAL INFECTIONS

Julius Schachter

University of California, San Francisco
Building 30, Room 416
1001 Potrero Avenue
San Francisco, CA 94110

Although *Chlamydia trachomatis* is one of the most common sexually transmitted pathogens, it is not recognized to be a major cause of upper urinary tract infections (1). It is, however, appropriate to discuss this organism in the context of this symposium because it is an important genital tract pathogen and these infections may be associated with urethral signs and symptoms. The purpose of this review is to briefly discuss those clinical conditions where chlamydial infection of the urinary tract is important and to discuss the currently used diagnostic tests for correctly identifying these infections and how these tests can be used. Some of the newer tests that are appearing with the technologic revolution in diagnostic procedures will also be mentioned.

*C. trachomatis* is the most common recognized cause of nongonococcal urethritis (NGU) in men, but accurate laboratory diagnosis is not required for appropriate management of this condition. NGU is diagnosed on the basis of exclusion; i.e., rule out gonococcal urethritis by use of Gram stain of urethral swab or discharge (1). If intracellular diplococci are seen, an appropriate course of antimicrobials as recommended for gonorrhea should be used. If the intracellular diplococci are not seen, a presumptive diagnosis of NGU is made (cultures should still be performed using Thayer-Martin) and appropriate therapy for NGU is called for.

*C. trachomatis* also can cause lower urinary tract disease in the female. Although the cervix is the most commonly infected site, urethral infection does occur. The specific syndrome with which chlamydial infection can be associated -- the acute urethral syndrome -- may also be managed without accurate diagnosis of chlamydial infection. This syndrome, which involves acute dysuria and frequency, can be divided into subsets by determination of bacterial colony counts from urine and the detection of polymorphonuclear leukocytes in the urine (2). Cervical infection with *Chlamydia* has been associated with that subset of women who have sterile pyuria. Thus, here too, appropriate therapy can be given based on tests which do not directly identify a chlamydial infection.

Thus, it is clear that most of the symptomatic chlamydial infections involving the urethra can be managed on a presumptive basis. Obviously, if possible, one would like to establish an etiologic diagnosis and in that context, specific microbiologic tests are needed. It is also true, of course, that asymptomatic infections could only be detected by use of appropriate microbiologic methods. There are other settings where chlamydial diagnosis is needed. These include not only genital tract infections but diseases involving ocular infections in adults or infants or in pneumonia in infants less than 6 months of age. Because chlamydial infections are amenable to chemotherapy, the laboratory can play an important role in helping the clinician manage many of these conditions.

## LABORATORY DIAGNOSIS OF CHLAMYDIA TRACHOMATIS INFECTION

In general, the basic principles of diagnosing chlamydial infections are similar to those for diagnosis of other bacterial infections (3). Serology, however, plays no role in diagnosing chlamydial infection of the lower genital tract and will not be discussed here. Thus, the only two approaches that are feasible are the demonstration of the agent in smears collected from the involved site (cytology) or cultural methods for isolating the organism in the clinical specimen.

## CYTOLOGY

Standard procedures for demonstrating chlamydiae in clinical specimens have been based on the characteristic morphology of the intracellular colony of chlamydiae. Being obligatory intracellular bacteria, these organisms are restricted to an intracellular environment for their life cycle and during the growth process produce characteristic inclusions which can be seen by Giemsa or other appropriate stains. These techniques, however, are not sufficiently sensitive for use in diagnosing genital tract infections. In one early study only 15% of those men yielding the organism from the urethra had Giemsa-staining inclusions in their urethral scrapings (4). Fluorescent antibody techniques using polyclonal antibodies were also used to demonstrate inclusions and were more sensitive than Giemsa, but still were not as sensitive as isolation in tissue culture. Because the reagents were not commercially available, the use of the test was restricted to a few research laboratories.

In the recent past, however, fluorescein-conjugated monoclonal antibodies which react with a species-specific epitope in the elementary body (the chlamydial infectious particle) outer membrane have been made commercially available (5). One such reagent (called MicroTrak(TM)) does not seem to detect inclusions particularly well in the clinical specimen, but does stain the free elementary bodies. The monoclonal technology produces a reagent which is far cleaner (i.e., less nonspecific staining) than the previous polyclonal reagents. Thus, it is possible to see the small fluorescing particles (250-350 nm) and if they are round (the typical morphology of the EB) and fluoresce a brilliant green, they are accepted as elementary bodies. It is clear that the test requires an experienced microscopist who has been trained to recognize the characteristic morphology of the elementary body.

In one evaluation performed in symptomatic patients attending a clinic for sexually transmitted diseases, the test was shown to have an approximately 92% sensitivity and a 98% specificity, as compared to tissue culture. Other experience with this test has been presented at national meetings and in publications.

The early results in my laboratory that we obtained during an ongoing evaluation of the technique, have not been nearly as good as the published experience. We have been testing the specimens collected during screening of asymptomatic women. With those cervical swabs our findings are a sensitivity of approximately 70% compared to culture, with a specificity of approximately 96%. It is likely that the differences in sensitivity which we observe are due to differences in culture method (see below) and test population, as asymptomatic women would predictably have less organism in their specimens than one would expect from symptomatic individuals. In our hands the predictive value (prevalence of infection by culture, 13%) of a positive test has been 60-70%. Thus, it would seem that the test is not particularly well suited for screening for inapparent chlamydial infection in a low risk population. However, the test could well play a role in diagnosis of chlamydial infections in settings where high rates of chlamydial infection exist, such as in individuals attending a clinic for sexually transmitted diseases or in high risk adolescent females attending inner city clinics where chlamydial infection rates of 15-40% have been documented (6, 7).

CULTURE METHODS

The standard procedure for isolating C. trachomatis uses McCoy cells. Although other cells that are also susceptible (HeLa, BHK-21, BMG, or L cells) may be substituted, most laboratories use the McCoy line and the improvements and modifications have been based on that cell line.

Because C. trachomatis does not grow well in cell culture, the infections have been enhanced by the use of centrifugation to improve the contact between the cells and the organism. Better chlamydial growth is obtained with the use of antimetabolites which restrict the metabolic processes of the host cell while allowing bacterial metabolism to proceed unchecked, thus giving chlamydiae an advantage in the intracellular environment. The procedures that have evolved include centrifugation of the clinical specimen for approximately 1 hour at 3,000 g at ambient (or preferably at 33-35 C) temperatures. The standard technique calls for use of 1-dram vials with approximately 12-13 mm coverslips supporting the monolayer of McCoy cells and the incubation is carried out in the presence of cycloheximide (8). Transport media generally used are either 2SP or tissue culture medium containing antibiotics to inhibit the growth of unwanted bacteria that are commonly found in the sites that chlamydiae infect. A typical antimicrobial mixture would include gentamycin at 10 ug/ml, vancomycin at 50 ug/ml and two to four units of fungizone per ml. Inoculated monolayers are incubated at 35 C for 2-3 days and examined for the presence of chlamydiae.

Ultimately, diagnosis of chlamydial infection is still based on microscopy. Characteristic inclusions must be demonstrated in the inoculated cell monolayer. Popular techniques include the use of Giemsa or iodine stain. Giemsa stain is not recommended on a routine basis because of problems in contrast with the cell monolayer. It may be difficult to differentiate inclusions during scanning of the monolayers. English workers have used darkfield microscopy of Giemsa stained monolayers (9). By this technique the elementary bodies and inclusions appear yellowish against a darker background and the monolayers may be more easily scanned. The iodine stain is the least sensitive procedure but is also the simplest technique available. It is based on the fact that the C. trachomatis inclusion contains glycogen and the inclusion will stain brown against a yellowish background of cell material. The most sensitive procedure for demonstrating inclusions in tissue culture involves use of fluorescent antibody technology. The above mentioned fluorescein-conjugated monoclonal antibodies have been extensively evaluated for staining inclusions in cell culture and have been shown to be more sensitive than the techniques based on light microscopy (10).

Modifications of the procedures outlined above include the use of

96-well, flat-bottomed microtiter plates, which will allow processing of larger numbers of specimens but provide a lessened cell area for

Table 1. Comparison of Isolation Methods

| Method (all blind pass) | % isolates obtained* |
|---|---|
| 1 - 96 well plate -- iodine | 48 |
| 2 - 96 well plate -- FA | 73 |
| 3 - vials -- iodine | 92 |

*cervical screening, asymptomatic population, 48/618 (7.8%) positive in any of the three methods.

infection (11). Blind passage of negative specimens will improve the sensitivity of the cell culture procedure. In highly positive specimens with large quantities of organism, the varying techniques are essentially equivalent, as most of the specimens will be positive on the first passage and there are adequate amounts of agent available to assure infection in the smaller cell population in the 96-well plates. However, in screening asymptomatic infections where lower amounts of agent are present, marked differences in sensitivity may be observed. The disparate results seen are almost always based on specimens that have less than 20 inclusions per coverslip in the first passage in vials. A representative comparison of the use of the 96-well plate stained by iodine or fluorescent antibody (FA) and the effect of a blind passage are presented in Table 1.

It is clear that the current state of the art approach for diagnosing chlamydial infection of the genital tract would use vials, fluorescein-conjugated monoclonal antibody to detect inclusions and a blind passage if the initial evaluated monolayer was found to be negative.

EMERGING METHODOLOGY

Other nonculture methods for diagnosing chlamydial infection are in the developmental stage. Enzyme immunoassay for detecting C. trachomatis antigen in genital tract specimens (Chlamydiazyme,(TM) Abbott Laboratories), is commercially available (12). The only published experience suggests that it is approximately 85% as sensitive as culture and approximately 98% specific.

Chlamydiae do not show DNA homology with any other microorganisms and this has been exploited in tests aimed at detecting chlamydial DNA in clinical specimens. Both plasmid and chromosomal DNA probes have been used (13, 14). These tests have been based on use of radiolabeled nucleic acid and until nonradioactive methods of detecting hybridization (such as biotin-avidin-conjugated enzyme systems) become available, these tests will not be practical.

EVALUATION OF NONCULTURE METHODS OF DIAGNOSIS

The variability of sensitivity observed in the different tissue culture methods will play a role in the assessment of nonculture methods of diagnosis. For example, the use of direct antigen detection procedures either by enzyme immunoassay or the fluorescein-conjugated monoclonal antibody will ultimately be based on comparison with culture. If the culture method is a less sensitive one, then obviously the nonculture method will appear to be relatively sensitive compared to the culture method. If, in fact, the nonculture method is more sensitive than culture, it will spuriously appear to have false-positive results because it will be detecting positives that are missed in culture. Unfortunately there are real false-positives in these tests, and their impact becomes more pronounced as the prevalence of infection decreases. Just as there are hazards in missing true positives, there are risks in the mislabel the test places on the false positive. Thus it is imperative that we have an accurate assessment of test performance, to know how to use the new tests.

In evaluating the literature it is imperative that the reader be aware of the population being tested and whether it is a population likely to have high or low amounts of agent in the clinical specimen and whether or not the culture method used was the most sensitive one available. One must also be aware that the most sensitive culture method is not 100% sensitive, as repeated evaluation of untreated positive individuals shows scattered failures to confirm the positive result (which then may be confirmed on a third or fourth test). It is likely that the best culture method available is only 80-90% sensitive in detecting chlamydial infection.

REFERENCES


1. Schachter, J. N. Engl. J. Med. 298:428,490 & 540. (1978).
2. Stamm, W.E., K.F. Wagner, R. Amsel, E.R. Alexander, M. Turck, G.W. Counts and K.K. Holmes. N. Engl. J. Med. 303:409. (1980).
3. Schachter, J. In: E. H. Lennette (ed.), Manual of Clinical Microbiology. p. 357. American Society for Microbiology: Washington, D.C. (1980).
4. Schachter, J. and C.R. Dawson. In: K. K. Holmes and D. Hobson (ed.), Nongonococcal Urethritis and Related Infections. p. 337. American Society for Microbiology: Washington, D.C. (1977).
5. Tam, M.R., W.E. Stamm, H.H. Handsfield, R. Stephens, C.C. Kuo, K.K. Holmes, K. Ditzenberger, M. Crieger, and R.C. Nowinski. N. Engl. J. Med. 310:1146. (1984).
6. Shafer, M.A., B. Blain, A. Beck, P. Dole, C.E. Irwin, R. Sweet and J. Schachter. J. Ped. 104:141. (1984).
7. Hardy, P.H., J.B. Hardy, E.E. Nell, D.A. Graham, M.R. Spence and R.C. Rosenbaum. Lancet 2(8398):333. (1984).
8. Ripa, K.T. and P-A. Mardh. J. Clin. Microbiol. 6:328. (1977).
9. Darougar, S., J.R. Kinnison and B.R. Jones. In: R. L. Nichols (ed.), Trachoma and Related Disorders Caused by Chlamydial Agents. p. 63. Excerpta Medica: Amsterdam. (1971).
10. Stamm, W.E., M. Tam, M. Koester and L. Cles. J. Clin. Microbiol. 17(4):666. (1983).
11. Yoder, B.L., W.E. Stamm, M.C. Koester and E.R. Alexander. J. Clin. Microbiol. 13(6):1036. (1981).
12. Schachter, J., W.M. McCormack, R.F. Smith, R.M. Parks, R. Bailey and A.C. Ohlin. J. Clin. Microbiol. 19:57. (1984).
13. Falkow, S. Presented paper at the International Society for STD Research 5th International Meeting, August 1-3, 1983, Seattle, Washington. (1983).
14. Palva, A., H. Jousimies-Somer, P. Saikku, P. Vaananen, H. Soderlund, and M. Ranki. FEMS Microbiol. Lett. 23(1984):83. (1984).

CHLAMYDIA TRACHOMATIS

Michael R. Spence and Joan F. Adler

Department of Obstetrics and Gynecology
Hahnemann University School of Medicine
Philadelphia, Pennsylvania 19102

Alexandria, Egypt sits on the Mediterranean coast of North Africa. It was in this city that the Rosetta Stone was found. The Rosetta Stone, a tabloid written in both ancient Greek and hieroglyphics, enabled the secrets of the pyramids to be unlocked. Upon translation of the writings of ancient Egypt, it was determined that an infectious urethritis was known approximately 3,000 years before Christ. This condition was contagious, was felt to be sexually transmitted, and a form of therapy which involved the intraurethral instillation of sandalwood oil was described. In Chapter 15 of Leviticus, which was written approximately 800 years BC, a contagious urethritis was also described. In these writings it was noted that this condition was contagious, was transmitted between man and woman, and necessitated the isolation of the infected person. Scholars feel that these writings describe a sexually transmitted disease caused by Neisseria gonorrhoeae. However, these may be some of the earliest writings describing nonspecific or nongonococcal urethritis. One of the major organisms associated with this particular condition is Chlamydia trachomatis. Since Chlamydia trachomatis is hyperendemic in the Middle East, it is quite possible that the urethritis that is described was caused by this agent.

Chlamydia trachomatis is a bacterium. It differs from many other bacteria in that it is an obligate intracellular parasite and requires an outside energy source. It cannot be grown on artificial media. Hence, it is necessary to cultivate this organism in a tissue culture system. The organism contains both RNA and DNA and divides by binary fission. The primary infectious particle, called the elementary body, invades the cell, multiplies and increases in size to become a reticulate body. After a finite number of the organisms inhabit a cell, the cell is lysed and the primary infectious agent, the elementary body, is released to infect adjacent cells, reinitiating the cycle. The organism has a predilection for columnar tissue, and similar to the gonococcus, is highly infectious for the genital tract and the eye.

There are many serovars of Chlamydia trachomatis that are infectious for man. The epidemiology of the infection, however, is dependent upon the serovar in question (1). Serotypes A, B, Ba and C are responsible for hyperendemic trachoma, a disease found in the Middle East that is associated with eye infections that can lead to subsequent blindness. Serotypes L1, L2, and L3 are responsible for lymphogranuloma venereum.

This is a sexually transmitted disease (STD) that is predominately found in subtropical climates. It initiates as a small ulcerative lesion on the external genitalia and is subsequently associated with significant lymphadenopathy and bubo formation.

The Chlamydia trachomatis infections that have come to the attention of both the scientific as well as the lay communities, however, are caused by serotypes D through K. These infections have earned Chlamydia the dubious honor of being one of the most common sexually transmitted pathogens.

There are many syndromes associated with Chlamydia trachomatis infections excluding trachoma and lymphogranuloma venereum. In the male patient, these include nongonococcal urethritis and epididymitis. Nongonococcal urethritis (a condition that is diagnosed by ruling out the presence of Neisseria gonorrhoeae as the cause of the urethral discharge) has been noted to be associated with Chlamydia trachomatis in up to 60% of cases. There are undoubtedly other microorganisms that are responsible for this condition, but Chlamydia is thought to be the major responsible organism. Another condition found in male patients secondary to Chlamydia is epididymitis. Although Neisseria gonorrhoeae is known to cause epididymitis, cases that were heretofore described as "idiopathic" epididymitis have now been demonstrated to be, on occasion, associated with Chlamydia trachomatis. Berger and his associates, through transscrotal aspirations of the epididymis, were able to demonstrate this organism as causative when Neisseria gonorrhoeae could not be isolated from the urethras of men with epididymitis (2).

In women, the urethral syndrome as described by Stamm and associates is a common cause of dysuria in a patient that has neither pyuria nor bacteriuria (3). Mucopurulent cervicitis has also been described in association with Chlamydia. It is a condition associated with a mucopurulent discharge from the cervix and friable ectopy. The role of Chlamydia trachomatis in Pelvic Inflammatory Disease is currently unclear. However, Scandinavian investigators have demonstrated that the organism can be isolated from the upper genital tract of women with this syndrome (4). It has been less often found in patients with Pelvic Inflammatory Disease in this country.

Two conditions that affect the newborn offspring of women with Chlamydia trachomatis infections in their cervices include ophthalmitis and pneumonia. The ophthalmitis is usually delayed in onset and mild in nature. Pneumonitis, as described by Beem and associates, is also a mild, slowly progressive problem in the neonate (5).

Other conditions that are thought to be associated with Chlamydia trachomatis that have been less well-substantiated include postpartum and postabortal endometritis. Additionally, some authors have described adverse pregnancy outcomes such as prematurity, stillbirth, and low birth weight infants as being associated with this organism. Further study is needed to substantiate these latter associations.

## CLINICAL DIAGNOSIS

Nongonococcal urethritis is an extremely common syndrome. The majority of cases are thought to be caused by Chlamydia trachomatis. The diagnosis of urethritis is based on the presence of dysuria and a urethral discharge. Severity of the symptoms is quite variable. The dysuria can be minimal and only associated with intermittent discomfort; or there can be frequent urination and a great deal of pain. Likewise, the discharge can be minimal and associated only with early morning rising, or can be profuse and purulent. It has been thought by many that the urethral discharge and dysuria associated with Neisseria gonorrhoeae was much different than that caused by Chlamydia. However, this is not the case. Both Neisseria gonorrhoeae and Chlamydia trachomatis can cause a very minimal, watery discharge or a very profuse, purulent discharge. Likewise, either agent can be associated with a significant degree of urethral discomfort. Hence, one has to use laboratory support methods to rule out Neisseria gonorrhoeae before the diagnosis of nongonococcal urethritis can be made. Likewise, chlamydial epididymitis can only be diagnosed by first ruling out Neisseria gonorrhoeae as the causative agent. This is particularly true since both agents are found in the same patient in up to 14% of the cases.

In the woman, acute urethral syndrome manifesting as a severe dysuria is often caused by Chlamydia trachomatis. Again, this is a diagnosis in which a bacterial agent must be ruled out rather than the ruling in of Chlamydia as the most common cause. Another entity that is frequently encountered in women is mucopurulent cervicitis. This diagnosis is made by noting the presence of a mucopurulent discharge coming from the endocervical canal with an attendant ectopy that is friable to touch (6). Neisseria gonorrhoeae can be responsible for this latter condition as well. Only after laboratory methods have ruled out this particular pathogen as causative, can one relate the problem to Chlamydia trachomatis. Pelvic Inflammatory Disease has also been described as either being gonococcal or nongonococcal. Scandinavian investigators have substantiated that the overwhelming majority of nongonococcal Pelvic Inflammatory Disease patients are infected with Chlamydia trachomatis (7). Although similar findings may be present in this country, this has yet to be substantiated.

The most common presentation of genitourinary Chlamydia trachomatis in the female is that of an asymptomatic infection. Although one can see the clinical presentations as described above, more commonly the patient harboring this particular organism has a perfectly normal-appearing lower genital tract. It is the exception rather than the rule that one finds evidence of a clinical syndrome when Chlamydia trachomatis is isolated.

The ophthalmitis that affects the newborn is usually insidious in onset, is somewhat delayed and usually does not occur until about a week after birth. This syndrome is rarely diagnosed in the newborn nursery, by either the Pediatrician or the Obstetrician/Gynecologist. More commonly it is the Emergency Room physician, private Pediatrician or the Ophthalmologist that sees this child and makes the diagnosis. These children are usually brought into the Emergency Room at 10-14 days of life because of a swollen eye or purulent discharge. If Chlamydia is suspected, a scraping of the conjunctiva can be stained with Giemsa stain to make a diagnosis. Pneumonia caused by Chlamydia trachomatis also is very insidious in onset. This condition usually begins between three and six weeks of life and is a mild lower respiratory disease manifested by an increased respiratory rate and a dry cough. The diagnosis is generally made by typical clinical picture and radiographs.

## LABORATORY DIAGNOSIS

The gold standard for the diagnosis of Chlamydia trachomatis is a culture. However, since this technique requires live cells, it is not readily available and quite often expensive. For this reason, the cost-effectiveness of this method must be questioned. Recently there have been numerous efforts to define a rapid, simple and inexpensive method of diagnosis. This has resulted in the development of rapid diagnostic tests as well as reevaluation of existing clinical materials and tests for the presence of clues that would lead to the diagnosis. There are fluorescent antibody techniques currently available which employ monoclonal antibody to Chlamydia trachomatis that are labeled with fluorescein isothiocyanate. Specimens obtained from the infected tissues are fixed and then stained with the monoclonal antibody that is labeled. They are then viewed under a fluorescent microscope. The presence of elementary bodies from Chlamydia results in an apple-green staining of these structures. This method is extremely sensitive and in trained hands can readily lead to the diagnosis of the organism. Other diagnostic methods employing color indicator change enzyme-linked immunosorbent assays (ELISA) have also been developed.

Work that we have conducted with one of the commercially available fluorescent antibody techniques has demonstrated a 90% specificity (8). The positive predictive value as well as the negative predictive value have both exceeded 90%. We, therefore, are very supportive of this as a technique for the rapid and inexpensive diagnosis of Chlamydia infections. In comparing our methods, we utilize a microwell technique as described by Stamm for culture (9). If one uses a more sensitive culture technique, such as the shell vial, one would anticipate that the sensitivity and specificity might be somewhat less. Nonetheless, we feel that we will probably identify approximately 80% of all infected patients. We also compared Papanicolaou smears as a diagnostic technique to both the fluorescent antibody technique and culture. Our data indicated that the Papanicolaou smear is neither sensitive nor specific, and at this time, we feel that the diagnosis of "cytopathologic changes consistent with Chlamydia" that is made by the cytopathologist is not only misleading, but potentially dangerous. These interpretations could result in the unnecessary employment of therapy in a patient which could have dire consequences.

In theory, the most reliable means of diagnosis is culture. This technique employs either irradiated McCoy cells or cycloheximide treated McCoy cells. These cells are then inoculated with clinical material and subsequently become infected. The sites of infectivity can be identified by employing either an iodine stain that will identify a brown inclusion, or by using the fluorescent antibody method. Recent work has demonstrated that DNA probes that are specific for Chlamydia trachomatis DNA can also be used and are a very sensitive indicator for infected cells. The major problem with using culture as a diagnostic method is the expense involved. The method requires a continual source of tissue culture cells, and in addition, the culture itself can take up to seven days before yielding a positive result. Additionally, once the cell culture has been infected, the infected site must be identified employing reagents and microscopy. The pros and cons of the various diagnostic methods are discussed elsewhere in these proceedings.

## THERAPY

Once the clinical diagnosis of Chlamydia is made, and it has been substantiated by laboratory methods, therapy is initiated. However, since adequate, affordable laboratory tests are not generally available, all to often the therapy is initiated on the basis of a diagnosis by exclusion. That is to say Neisseria gonorrhoeae is ruled out and an assumption made that the causative organism is Chlamydia trachomatis. Hence, a large number of patients are treated for Chlamydia infections without the diagnosis being supported by laboratory techniques. The current treatments of choice include tetracycline hydrochloride and erythromycin. Other substituted tetracyclines have been shown to be equally as effective. Current therapy involves treating the patient for a minimum of seven days and some regimens require up to 14 days. These regimens were reviewed in the Morbidity and Mortality Weekly Report of 22 August 1982.

There is always a question as to whether or not to treat an asymptomatic patient. Certainly if one is dealing with an individual with symptoms, an asymptomatic sexual partner should be treated. However, to treat all asymptomatic harborers of Chlamydia trachomatis is quite difficult. This would require identification of the population. To identify the asymptomatic host could require extensive screening. The employment of an expensive technique for screening large populations is probably not cost-effective. If screening methods are to be employed to identify infected patients then at-risk populations should be sought. These include sexually active teenagers, especially those 17 years of age and below. Screening the entire population does not make sense because the risk of infection is quite variable depending upon the population evaluated.

In summary, Chlamydia trachomatis appears to have been around for many years, if not centuries. The organism is associated with a myriad of clinical conditions. The diagnosis is usually based on the presence of specific syndromes and ruling out other pathogens. The most common situation, however, is an asymptomatic patient. There are rapid, simple, and inexpensive diagnostic methods available. However, the more accurate techniques are expensive. Once the organism is identified, the patient can be treated with antimicrobial agents which can result in cure. Current problems include identifying the at-risk groups for infection, and determining the significance of asymptomatically harboring the organism.

REFERENCES


1. J. Schachter: Chlamydial Infections, Part I. N. Engl. J. Med. 298:428-435, 1978.
2. R.E. Berger: Urethritis and epididymitis. Semin Urol. 1:121-129, 1983.
3. W. Stamm, K.F. Wagner et al: Causes of the Acute Urethral Syndrome in Women. N. Engl. J. Med. 303:409-415, 1980.
4. P.A. Mardh, K.T. Ripa et al: Chlamydia trachomatis infection in patients with acute salpingitis. N. Engl. J. Med. 296:1377-1379, 1977.
5. M.D. Beem, E.M. Saxon: Respiratory tract colonization and a distinctive pneumonia syndrome in infants infected with Chlamydia trachomatis. N. Eng. J. Med. 296:306-310, 1977.
6. E. Rees, I.A. Tait, D. Hobson et al: Chlamydia in relation to cervical infection and PID, nongonococcal urethritis and related infections. Edited by K.K. Holmes, D. Hobson. Washington, D.C., Amer. Soc. for Microbiol., 1977, pp. 67-76.
7. K.T. Ripa et al: Chlamydia trachomatis infection in patients with laparoscopically verified acute salpingitis. A. J. Obstet. Gynecol. 138:960-964, 1980.
8. W.E. Stamm, H.R. Harrison et al: Diagnosis of Chlamydia trachomatis infections by direct immunofluorescence staining of genital secretions. Annals of Int. Med. 101:638-641, 1984.
9. W.E. Stamm, M. Tam, M. Koester, L. Cles: Detection of Chlamydia trachomatis inclusions in McCoy cell cultures with fluorescein conjugated monoclonal antibodies. J. Clin. Microbiol. 17:666-668, 1983.

# THE DEFINITIVE DIAGNOSIS OF MYCOPLASMA INFECTIONS

Ruth B. Kundsin

Brigham and Women's Hospital
Department of Microbiology and Molecular Genetics
Harvard Medical School, Boston, MA 02115

*Mycoplasma pneumoniae* is no longer the only mycoplasma recognized as a pathogen for humans. The emergence of *Mycoplasma hominis* and *Ureaplasma urealyticum* as genitourinary tract pathogens in adults (1), as well as for the fetus in utero and the neonate (2), makes isolation of these organisms no longer a research exercise but an essential diagnostic laboratory test. It is for this reason that the methodology for isolation and identification of these organisms must be reviewed. Another area of major import has been the development of a reproducible antibiotic susceptibility test which has relevance to attainable serum levels of the different antibiotics. This is critical for instituting appropriate and effective therapy.

Too long have patients been treated empirically depending on the clinician's intuition and prejudice.

## LABORATORY DIAGNOSIS

### Specimens

The most common specimens are urine and cervical swabs in the female, and urine, semen, and urethral swabs in the male. Two specimens from each patient are usually submitted. Other specimens can be amniotic fluid, tissue from an endometrial biopsy, products of conception, and tissue or swabs obtained at the time of surgery by the obstetrician or gynecologist. Most commonly, with female patients, the clinician takes the cervical swab and the patient brings it to the laboratory and at the same time produces a urine specimen. The male patients are instructed to take their own urethral specimen in the laboratory prior to voiding.

If specimens are transported any distance, requiring more than one hour of travel, swabs should be placed in 0.5 ml of normal saline. Both *U. urealyticum* and *M. hominis* survive for longer periods in normal saline than in distilled water at room temperature. In urine both *U. urealyticum* and *M. hominis* can survive for days. If specimens are mailed however, saline for the swabs is essential and all specimens including urine or urine sediment should be packed in dry ice prior to shipping. Freezing results in a substantial loss of organisms and should only be used as a last resort.

PROCESSING OF SPECIMENS

The urine (15 ml) is spun down in a clinical centrifuge for ten minutes. The supernatant (14 ml) is discarded and the remaining one milliliter is used for culture. If enough specimen is available, the remainder is spun and the sediment is frozen for use as a backup in the event the test is equivocal, or for antibiotic susceptibility testing if the culture is positive and the clinician requests it.

Both the genital specimen and the urine sediment are streaked on Shepard's A7 agar (3), and each (the original swab and .05 ml of urine sediment) is also placed into Boston Broth (4). If a culturette type of plastic container has been sent with the swab, broth is poured into the container. Mucus which adheres to the sides of the container is a good source of genital mycoplasmas. The agar plate is sealed using the Fortner technique (5). Any other technique for anaerobic incubation is equally satisfactory. All media are incubated at 36°C and observed as follows. Broths are observed daily for a color change. The change in color from yellow to pink is usually detected early at the bottom of the tube and gradually moves up. Subcultures are negative when the contents of the whole tube have become alkaline. The agar medium is scanned at 48 hours and daily thereafter. If there is any doubt about the colonies on the solid agar, subcultures should be made when the broth medium is just starting to turn color. A specimen is reported as positive only when typical colonies are seen on the agar plate. The broth serves only to flag the specimen as positive. Confirmation is made by visualizing colonies on agar.

Ureaplasmas form dark brown colonies due to the manganese salts in the medium. Classical mycoplasmas exhibit no color on this medium. They can be stained by means of the Dienes stain. Ureaplasmas need no further identification, classical mycoplasmas do. In our experience the only classical mycoplasma we have found in the genitourinary tract is M. hominis. There have been reports of isolations of other mycoplasmas and for that reason positive identification must be done using M. hominis antisera in the growth inhibition test (6).

RESULTS OF ISOLATIONS

The patients referred to our laboratory fall into two categories. They either have an active infection or a history of infertility. The infertility patients are usually asymptomatic, while the patients with infection have some symptom such as discharge, urinary frequency, burning on urination, or lower quadrant pain.

Table 1 compares isolations from female patients with histories of infertility and from female patients with infection. The genital mycoplasmas were isolated from 61% of infertility patients, and from 50% of patients with infection. The difference is statistically significant (P=.01) and is due to the rate of isolation of ureaplasmas, the predominant isolate. M. hominis isolations remained the same in both groups, 8.6% and 9%. Because 50% of patients with infection did not yield a mycoplasma, other microorganisms should be sought. In addition to routine bacteriology, cultures should be done specifically for chlamydiae and gonococci.

Table 2 compares isolations from male patients. In male patients the difference in isolation rates from infertility patients and patients with infection was not statistically significant when both genital mycoplasmas were considered (P=.45). What was noteworthy was that M. hominis

TABLE 1. FEMALE PATIENTS WITH HISTORY OF INFERTILITY AND INFECTION (January thru December 1983)

| | Infertility No. | Percent | Infection No. | Percent |
|---|---|---|---|---|
| Ureaplasma urealyticum | 815 | (52%) | 60 | (41%) |
| Ureaplasma urealyticum and Mycoplasma hominis | 118 | ( 8%) | 14 | ( 9%) |
| Mycoplasma hominis | 10 | (.6%) | 0 | |
| Any Mycoplasma* | 943 | (61%) | 74 | (50%) |
| No Mycoplasma | 610 | (39%) | 74 | (50%) |
| Total | 1553 | | 148 | |

* Any mycoplasma - Infertility vs. Infection $X^2 = 6.46$ $P = .01$

TABLE 2. MALE PATIENTS WITH HISTORY OF INFERTILITY AND INFECTION (January thru December 1983)

| | Infertility No. | Percent | Infection No. | Percent |
|---|---|---|---|---|
| Ureaplasma urealyticum | 69 | (37%) | 29 | (35%) |
| Ureaplasma urealyticum and Mycoplasma hominis | 5 | ( 3%) | 7 | ( 8%) |
| Mycoplasma hominis | 1 | (.5%) | 1 | ( 1%) |
| Any Mycoplasma* | 75 | (40%) | 37 | (45%) |
| No Mycoplasma | 114 | (60%) | 46 | (55%) |
| Total | 189 | | 83 | |

*Any mycoplasma - Infertility vs. Infection $X^2 = .57$ $P = .45$ (not significant)

isolations did differ significantly (P=.03) between the two types of patients, with isolations of 9% from the patients with infection and 3% from patients with infertility. When male and female patients are compared in the two categories, another interesting observation can be made. Female patients with infertility had a significantly higher rate of isolation of both U. urealyticum and M. hominis than male patients. Not so, with patients with infection. In that group no significant difference could be found in isolation rates of the genital mycoplasmas between males and females. This is shown in Table 3.

Table 4 shows the isolation rate of the genital mycoplamas from semen. The rate of isolation is lower than that from infertility patients and patients with infection. This is due to the inclusion of healthy donors in the tested group. Donors of semen for artificial insemination are screened for genital mycoplasmas prior to the procedure. These are healthy, asymptomatic young men and one would not expect a high isolation rate from them. Ureaplasmas again are the predominant isolates.

TABLE 3. COMPARISON OF FEMALE AND MALE PATIENTS WITH HISTORY OF INFERTILITY AND INFECTION
(January thru December 1983)

| | Infertility | | Infection | |
|---|---|---|---|---|
| | Female | Male | Female | Male |
| Ureaplasma urealyticum | 815 (52%) | 69 (37%) | 60 (41%) | 29 (35%) |
| | P = .00003 | | P = .40 | |
| Ureaplasma urealyticum and Mycoplasma hominis | 118 (8%) | 5 (3%) | 14 (9%) | 7 (8%) |
| | P = .012 | | P = .79 | |
| Mycoplasma hominis | 10 (.6%) | 1 (.5%) | 0 | 1 (1%) |
| | P = .85 | | | |
| Any Mycoplasma | 943 (61%) | 75 (40%) | 74 (50%) | 37 (45%) |
| | P = .00000003 | | P = .43 | |
| Negative | 610 (39%) | 114 (60%) | 74 (50%) | 46 (55%) |
| Total | 1553 | 189 | 148 | 83 |

TABLE 4. UREAPLASMA UREALYTICUM AND MYCOPLASMA HOMINIS IN SEMEN (327 Specimens)

| | No. | Percent |
|---|---|---|
| Negative | 227 | (69%) |
| Positive* | 100 | (31%) |
| *Ureaplasma urealyticum | 93 | (28%) |
| Ureaplasma urealyticum and Mycoplasma hominis | 5 | (1.5%) |
| Mycoplasma hominis | 2 | (0.6%) |
| Total Positive | 100 | |

We encourage the submission of two specimens from each patient. Two specimens assure a better chance of recovery of the genital mycoplasmas. Although in general, cultures from the genital tract and the urine have shown agreement in 88% of 659 female patients, and 86% of 66 male patients. When non-agreement has occurred, the urine was positive and the genital culture was negative, except in 2% of female patients in whom cervical cultures were positive and urine was negative. Semen was a good specimen as it was always in agreement with other specimens from the male patient. When only one specimen can be obtained, urine from the female, and semen from the male are the optimal specimens.

In a study of the placentas of 802 newborns (2), placental cultures were found retrospectively to show good correlation with pregnancy outcome. Isolations of genital mycoplasmas were found to be related significantly to low birthweight, low gestational age, and admission to the intensive care unit (2). A placental culture obviously could not be taken prior to delivery. All correlations in the study were made following birth. Chorioamnionitis was also found to be correlated with the isolation of the genital mycoplasmas from the placenta.

The implications are that colonization of the genital tract of both males and females with genital mycoplasmas affords an opportunity for these microorganisms to gain access to the upper female genital tract and to adversely affect pregnancy outcome.

THERAPY

Antibiotic susceptibility testing is essential for initiating appropriate therapy. The broth-disk method (7) is the simplest method, and is well correlated with the results of antibiotic therapy. Urine sediment (.05 ml) is used for inoculating tubes of broth containing antibiotics in concentrations approximating attainable serum levels.

Table 5 shows results of susceptibility tests of U. urealyticum and M. hominis strains isolated from patients. Of 523 strains of ureaplasmas, 53(10%) were found to be resistant to all tetracyclines. An additional 4% were found resistant to at least one tetracycline. Of 158 M. hominus isolates, 11% were found resistant to all tetracyclines, 22% were partially resistant. Treatment of patients carrying resistant strains has presented a problem, particularly with ureaplasma infections. All M. hominis isolates to date have been found susceptible to clindamycin so that a satisfactory alternative to the tetracyclines is available for use.

TABLE 5. SUSCEPTIBILITIES OF U. UREALYTICUM AND M. HOMINIS TO FOUR TETRACYCLINES+

DOXYCYCLINE (1 UG/ML, MINOCYCLINE (1 UG/ML)
DEMECLOCYCLINE (1 UG/ML), TETRACYCLINE (6 UG/ML)

| RESULTS | U. UREALYTICUM 523 STRAINS | | M. HOMINIS 158 STRAINS | |
|---|---|---|---|---|
| SUSCEPTIBLE TO ALL | 448 | (86%) | 106 | (67%) |
| RESISTANT TO ALL | 53 | (10%) | 17 | (11%) |
| PARTIALLY SUSCEPTIBLE* | 22 | ( 4%) | 35 | (22%) |

*Resistant to at least one tetracycline.
+ Broth-disk method

**Other antibiotics which have been tested against resistant ureaplasmas are shown in Table 6. While chloramphenicol, streptomycin, kanamycin, and gentamicin, have been shown by in-vitro testing to be effective in inhibiting some tetracycline resistant strains of the genital mycoplasmas, clinicians are reluctant to use them because of potentially adverse side reactions.**

TABLE 6. TETRACYCLINE RESISTANT STRAINS OF U. UREALYTICUM SUSCEPTIBILITIES TO OTHER ANTIBIOTICS*

| Antibiotic | | Susceptible No./Total | Susceptible Percent |
|---|---|---|---|
| Chloramphenicol | (6 ug/ml) | 13 / 17 | 76% |
| Streptomycin | (10 ug/ml) | 11 / 17 | 65% |
| Gentamicin | (4 ug/ml) | 6 / 24 | 25% |
| Kanamycin | (12 ug/ml) | 4 / 16 | 25% |

* Broth-disk method

The most recent attempt to treat tetracycline resistant ureaplasma infections has involved the use of acetohydroxamic acid in combination with erythromycin and doxycycline. In vitro testing is done first to determine whether the resistant strain is susceptible to 75 mcg. or less of acetohydroxamic acid in the presence of erythromycin and doxycycline in concentrations attainable in serum. With this combination, ureaplasmas have been eradicated from fifteen patients, both husband and wife of five couples with problems of infertility, and five women with infection. No side effects were reported by these patients. One couple achieved a successful pregnancy following treatment.

A major concern in this work had been that the increasing sophistication of the diagnostic laboratory has not been accompanied by an acceptance of the results by the practicing clinician. Working at the advancing edge of diagnostic medicine has taxed the communications between patients, clinician, and laboratory. The communication problem is exemplified by, four symptomatic women with persistent untreated genitourinary tract infections from whom genital mycoplasmas had been isolated who were referred to psychiatrists by their clinicians. This despite the formal recognition of these organisms as etiologic agents of nongonococcal urethritis in the male, and mounting evidence of their association with genitourinary tract infection in the female, resulting in infertility, spontaneous abortion, ectopic pregnancy, postpartum fever, and overt pelvic inflammatory disease.

REFERENCES

1. Clyde, W.A., Jr. Methods in Mycoplasmology Vol. II Academic Press (1983).
2. Kundsin, R.B., S.G. Driscoll, R.R. Monson, C. Yeh, S.A. Biano and W.D. Cochran. Association of Ureaplasma urealyticum In the Placenta with Perinatal Morbidity and Mortality. N.E.J. Med. 310: 941 (1984)
3. Shepard, M.C. and C.D. Lunceford. Differential Agar Medium (A&) for

Identification of Ureaplasma urealyticum (human T mycoplasmas) In Primary Culture of Clinical Material. J. Clin. Microbial. 3: 613 (1976).

4. Leland, D.S., M.A. Lapworth, R.B. Jones and M.L.V. French. Comparative Evaluation of Media for Isolation of Ureaplasma urealyticum and Genital Mycoplasma Species. J. Clinical Microbial. 16: 709 (1982).
5. Fortner, J.. A Simple Plating Method for Culture of Obligate Anaerobes. Zentrable. Bact. Parasit. Infekt. Hyg. 108: 55 (1928).
6. Clyde, W.A., Jr. Mycoplasma Species Identification Based Upon Growth Inhibition by Specific Antisera. J. Immunol. 92: 958 (1964).
7. Spaepen, M.S. and R.B. Kundsin. Simple, Direct Broth-Disk Method for Antibiotic Susceptibility Testing of Ureaplasma urealyticum. Antimicrob. Agents and Chemother. 11: 267 (1977).

# PATHOGENESIS AND SIGNIFICANCE OF UROGENITAL MYCOPLASMAL INFECTIONS

G.H. Cassell[1], J.K. Davis[2], K.B. Waites[13], P.T. Rudd[1], D. Talkington[1], D. Crouse[4], and S.A. Horowitz[1]

[1]Department of Microbiology, [2]Department of Comparative Medicine, [3]Department of Pathology and Spain Rehabilitation Center, [4]Department of Pediatrics University of Alabama Schools of Medicine and Dentistry University of Alabama at Birmingham, University Station Birmingham, Alabama 35294

Of the seven species of mycoplasmas isolated from the urogenital tract of humans, Ureaplasma urealyticum and Mycoplasma hominis are the ones found most commonly and are the only two known to cause disease (1-3). Mycoplasma genitalium is a newly identified species first isolated from males with urethritis (4-6). Serological studies of females with pelvic inflammatory disease (7) and experimental inoculation of primates (8-10) suggest that this organism may also be pathogenic for humans, although its prevalence is unknown.

U. urealyticum can be found in the cervix or vagina of 40-80% of sexually mature, asymptomatic women (1,2), and M. hominis in 21-53% (1-3). The incidence of each is somewhat lower in the urethra of normal males (1,2). In women, colonization is linked to younger age, lower socioeconomic status, sexual activity with multiple partners, black ethnicity, and oral contraceptive use (11). U. urealyticum and M. hominis may be transmitted to as many as 38% of babies born to infected mothers (12-14). Colonization of most infants appears to be transient with a sharp decline in isolation rates after 3 months of age. Less than 10% of older children and sexually inexperienced adults are colonized (1,2). Colonization after puberty increases with sexual activity (1,2).

Neither U. urealyticum nor M. hominis has been shown to cause disease in the lower genital tract of the female. In fact, these organisms are probably commensals in this site. Diseases for which they have been suspected to play an etiological role are listed in Table 1. All are either diseases of the upper genito-urinary tract in females or diseases of the male. The difficulty with accepting these organisms as the cause of disease in each has usually arisen from the fact that either cultural samples cannot be easily obtained from the affected site or that

Table I.

| Disease | References | Causative Agents: M. hominis | U. urealyticum |
|---|---|---|---|
| Urethritis of males | (15,16) | -[a] | + |
| Urethroprostatitis | (17,18) | - | +[b] |
| Female urethral syndrome | (19-21) | - | ± |
| Pyelonephritis | (22,24,25) | + | ± |
| Urinary calculi | (26-30) | - | + |
| Vaginitis | (1-3) | - | - |
| Cervicitis | (1-3) | - | - |
| Pelvic inflammatory disease | (31-34) | + | ± |
| Infertility | (1-3,35) | - | ± |
| Chorioamnionitis | (36-41) | ± | + |
| Spontaneous abortion | (1-3,38,40-43) | ± | ± |
| Prematurity/Low birth weight | (12,13,38,39,44-48) | - | ± |
| Intrauterine growth retardation | (38,39,44) | - | ± |
| Postpartum fever | (1-3) | + | ± |
| Congenital pneumonia | (37,41,49-53) | + | + |
| Respiratory distress in newborns | (54-57) | ± | ± |
| Meningitis in newborns | (58) | + | - |
| Abscesses in newborns | (59-61) | + | - |
| Extragenital disease in adults (including septic arthritis) | (61-64,76-79) | + | + |

a - = No association or causal role demonstrated

b + = Causal Role

c ± = Significant association, and/or strong suggestive evidence but causal role not proven.

the organisms can be recovered from the affected site in asymptomatic individuals.

Even in diseases where Koch's postulates have been fulfilled (i.e., M. hominis and pelvic inflammatory disease (PID)), attempts to link inflammatory lesions of the upper tract with cultural isolation from the lower tract have delayed recognition of the etiological significance of these organisms. Recent carefully controlled clinical studies and experimental infection of laboratory animals have shown the disease producing potential of both U. urealyticum and M. hominis. A major principle amply illustrated in these studies is that only in a subpopulation of individuals infected in the lower genitourinary tract do the organisms reach the upper tract and only in some of these individuals does disease ensue. In no instance have the factors that predispose to upper tract colonization or development of disease been delineated. In many of the diseases considered, these factors may be of more importance for the development of lesions than the organism involved. While U. urealyticum or M. hominis may be responsible for inflammatory lesions in some instances, they primarily appear to be opportunists and other microbes may induce nearly identical lesions in other individuals. Ultimately, understanding of the predisposing factors may prove of more benefit in controlling such conditions than the actual organisms isolated from the lesions.

## EVIDENCE THAT GENITAL MYCOPLASMAS INDUCE INFLAMMATION

Genital infection of the bovine species with Ureaplasma diversum offers interesting parallels with the role of U. urealyticum in humans. The former was thought to cause granular vulvitis in cows nearly two decades ago. However, not all animals with the organism had lesions; and proof that the lesions were directly linked to U. diversum required experimental inoculation of proven Ureaplasma free animals (80). Subsequently, U. diversum has been shown to induce mastitis (81), salpingitis (80), endometritis (80), spontaneous abortion (82,83), and neonatal calf pneumonia (82-84). In all of these diseases, proof of a causative role ultimately was achieved by inoculation of the organisms into gnotobiotic animals, or animals proven to be free of ureaplasmal infection. Obviously this approach cannot be taken with U. urealyticum, and while U. diversum probably is more pathogenic than U. urealyticum, as evidenced by induction of inflammatory lesions in the most common site of isolation, the parallels between the two organisms and especially between the early attempts to prove the role of U. diversum in bovine disease and the current situation in humans with U. urealyticum cannot be ignored.

Direct inoculation of M. hominis into the fallopian tubes of grivet monkeys produces a para-metritis and salpingitis (85). Ascending M. hominis infection in the monkeys must be preceded by mechanical injury of the epithelial barrier with subsequent spread occurring via blood and lymph vessels rather than by the canalicular route. In fallopian tube organ culture, M. hominis induces ciliary swelling but no other obvious pathological changes (86). Similar experiments with U. urealyticum in grivet monkeys and organ cultures were unsuccessful (87,88), but inoculation of the urethra of Macaca fascicularis males induced transient infections associated in some cases with urethritis (89). Evidence for the capability of U. urealyticum to induce inflammatory lesions in humans comes from experimental inoculation of the organism into the urethra of men (16). At doses of $5\times10^{4}$ organisms, fever, pyuria, and dysuria were induced along with a rise in specific antibody titers.

There are numerous individual reports demonstrating that both organisms can occasionally gain access to the blood stream. In the case of U. urealyticum, this has been reported solely from cases of post-abortal and post-partum septicemia (1-3). Septicemia due to M. hominis apparently occurs more frequently and has been demonstrated in a variety of conditions (62-64,66,69-75). In all of these, the predisposing cause could have been either catheterization of the bladder or lowered immune responsiveness due either to the underlying disease or iatrogenic immunosuppression.

The strongest evidence for the inflammatory capabilities of both U. urealyticum and M. hominis in humans comes from studies of hypogammaglobulinaemic individuals. In these individuals, M. hominis has produced arthritis (76) and U. urealyticum has produced not only arthritis but also subcutaneous abscesses (77-79) and persistent urethritis (90,91). While only a limited number of these patients have been studied, both organisms have been isolated in pure cultures from lesions, and the lesions responded to appropriate antibiotic treatment or specific hyperimmune serum. In at least one case, urethritis recurred several times and in each reoccurence antibiotic resistant ureaplasmas were isolated (90).

Given the above evidence, the capability of both organisms to induce lesions in humans must be accepted. Whether they do so in natural infection of normal individuals the frequency with which this occurs, the disease syndromes with which these organisms are associated, and the predisposing host factors involved are the critical questions that remain unanswered in many instances.

In a limited number of diseases, there is almost universal agreement that M. hominis or U. urealyticum are involved in the etiology. It should be noted that in most instances identical or similar lesions are induced by other bacteria, thus even though these organisms are involved, their relative importance is often unknown.

## DISEASES CAUSED BY GENITAL MYCOPLASMAS

Urinary Tract: Three conditions of the urinary tract definitively proven to be due to the genital mycoplasmas are urethritis in males due to *U. urealyticum* (15,16), urinary calculi due to ureaplasmas (26-30), and pyelonephritis caused by *M. hominis* (22).

While confusion still exists concerning the proportion of cases of nongonococcal urethritis due to ureaplasmas, the fact that it is responsible for some cases should no longer be disputed. Human (16) and animals (89,92) inoculation studies and the occurrence in immunodeficient patients (90) provide indisputable evidence. Carefully controlled antibiotic (93-95) and recent serological studies (96) are also supportive of a causal role. The common occurrence of ureaplasmas in the urethra of asymptomatic men suggest either that only certain serotypes of ureaplasmas are pathogenic or that predisposing factors, such as a lack of mucosal immunity, must exist in those individuals that do develop disease. Alternatively, disease may only develop upon initial exposure to these organisms. If so, study of individuals attending sexually transmitted disease clinics are not likely to provide useful information. Almost all studies to date have focused on these patients.

Urinary stones composed of struvite and carbonate-apatite account for 20% of all urinary tract stones (97) and are induced by the enzymatic breakdown of urea by bacterial urease which splits urea into ammonia and carbon dioxide. Proteus species and to a lesser extent Klebsiella, Pseudomonas, and Staphylococcus species are the usual causes in humans (98). However, *U. urealyticum* also produces urease, and has been demonstrated to induce crystallization of struvite and calcium phosphates *in vitro* in artificial urine (30) although the formation of crystals is slower with these organisms than with *Proteus mirabilis*, the most common cause of these stones in humans. Thus, their capability to induce stones in the appropriate location is proven. Renal calculi have been induced experimentally in rats by inoculation of pure cultures of *U. urealyticum* directly into the bladder and renal pelvis (28,29). *U. urealyticum* has been isolated from stones recovered by surgery in 6 of 15 patients (27). In four of these, no other urease producing organisms were isolated either in the stone or in urine sampled from the renal pelvis. The major remaining questions concerning the role of this organisms in production of urinary calculi is the frequency with which the organisms reaches the kidney, the predisposing factors that allow this to occur, and the relative frequency of renal calculi induced by this organism compared to those induced by other organisms.

Despite the high incidence of *M. hominis* in the lower urogenital tract, this organism has been isolated from the upper urinary tract only in patients with symptoms of acute infection (22) and in fact is isolated from the urine in 10% of these patients. In two studies (99,100), *M. hominis* was recovered from samples of urine collected from the upper urinary tract (ureters) during surgery or from ureteral catheterization from 7 (4 of which were in pure culture) of 80 patients with acute pyelonephritis and from 3 of 18 patients with acute exacerbation of chronic pyelonephritis. The organism was not found in the upper urinary tract of 22 patients with chronic pyelonephritis without acute exacerbation nor from 60 patients with non-infectious urinary tract disease. Ureaplasmas were isolated from the upper urinary tract of five patients but the isolation rate was not significantly different from that in the control group. In an additional cultural study of patients with acute urinary tract symptoms in which antibodies to M. hominis were found in the urine, the organism was isolated from the upper urinary tract in seven (101). Overall, M. hominis is thought to be involved in 5% of cases of acute pyelonephritis in humans. Interestingly, predisposing factors including obstruction or instrumentation of the urinary tract occur in about 50% of cases in which M. hominis is thought to be the etiological cause (22).

Genital Diseases: Only one entity of either the male or female genital tract has definitely been shown to be caused by the genital mycoplasmas. PID is an increasingly common disease of multifactorial etiology. PID can be caused iatrogenically or occur naturally from infections with various bacteria, the most common of which are Neisseria gonorrhoeae and Chlamydia trachomatis (102). Although the exact proportion of cases is unknown, M. hominis but not U. urealyticum is also a cause of PID (31-34). As stated earlier, inoculation of M. hominis into fallopian tubes of monkeys induces parametritis and salpingitis within 3 days (85), and inoculation of human fallopian tube explants produces ciliostasis (86). The organism has been isolated in pure cultures from the fallopian tubes of approximately 8% of women with salpingitis as diagnosed by laparoscopy as compared to 0% of women without lesions (31). The organisms can also be isolated from the endometrium. In addition, a role for these organisms in cases of PID not associated with either N. gonorrhoeae or C. trachomatis is supported by significant increases in specific antibody (33). While U. urealyticum has been isolated directly from affected fallopian tubes (34), it usually is found in the presence of other known pathogens. Furthermore, experimental animal inoculation (87) and fallopian tube organ culture (88) studies do not support a causal role.

Disorders of Reproduction: While M. hominis and U. urealyticum have been found to be associated with a number of disorders of reproduction, convincing evidence for a causative role exists for only chorioamnionitis. Isolation of U. urealyticum from the infant but not maternal cervix was found to be significantly associated with chorioamnionitis even when the data were stratified according to the infant's birth weight, length, head circumference, sex gestational age, placental weight, duration of labor and ruptured membranes, mother's race, language, number of prenatal visits, and smoking habits (104). Unfortunately this study did not assess the possible role of other etiologic agents. Three studies have assessed the relationship of mycoplasmal isolation from the placenta and the presence of chorioamnionitis (38-40). Two of these rigorously sought the presence of other fastidious microorganisms. In these, U. urealyticum alone was significantly associated with the presence of inflammation (39,40). The lesions were not associated with inflammation of the chorionic villi thus suggesting an ascending route of infection. While the placental studies took into account the time of membrane rupture, they did not consider the duration of labor nor the presence of U. urealyticum in the cervix/vagina of study and control patients. Recent evidence indicates that bacteria from the vagina and cervix often invade the amniotic fluid at the onset of labor and prior to membrane rupture (103-108). Risk of infection of the placenta with mycoplasmas also increases with rupture of the membranes, duration of labor, and number of vaginal exams (109,110). Although unlikely, the difference in U. urealyticum isolation from placentas between patient groups might be due to differences in the duration of labor and the ureaplasmal cervical carriage rate and/or differences in the number of organisms present.

The most convincing evidence that genital mycoplasmas can cause chorioamnionitis and only in subpopulation of individuals colonized in the lower tract comes from studies of intra-amniotic fluid infection. Up to 4% of fluids obtained by transabdominal amniocentesis are discolored due to apparent hemorrhage into the amniotic cavity (111,113). In approximately one-third of these cases, the pregnancy terminates in abortion, stillbirth, or early death of the neonate (114-115). In a recent study (37), M. hominis was isolated from two and U. urealyticum was isolated from two of 33 discolored fluids collected between the 16th and 20th week of pregnancy as compared to no isolations from 28 normal fluids obtained from women matched for cervicovaginal carriage of genital mycoplasmas, socioeconomic status, and indications for amniocentesis. Viruses, chlamydiae, and other bacteria were not isolated from either clear or discolored fluids. At the time of amniocentesis, no neutrophils were found in the amniotic fluid from either patient from which M. hominis was isolated, but were present in both fluids from which U. urealyticum was isolated. Ultimately, both of the patients from whom ureaplasmas were isolated delivered prematurely and both infants failed to survive. In both, severe chorioamnionitis, vasculitis, and funisitis were present in the placenta and immunofluorescence was used to localize U. urealyticum in the lesions (unpublished observations). U. urealyticum was isolated from the placenta in the absence of aerobic and strict anaerobic bacteria, chlamydiae, or viruses. Furthermore, following death of the infants, U. urealyticum was isolated in pure cultures from a variety of organs and tissues. While one isolate of M. hominis was obtained on the first attempt at amniocentesis, the other and the two ureaplasmal isolates were obtained following previous unsuccessful attempts to collect fluid. Thus the possibility that the ureaplasmas were introduced into the amniotic fluid by passage of the needle through the endometrium cannot be excluded. Regardless of the route of infection, the results do indicate that U. urealyticum in the absence of other microorganisms is capable of initiating an inflammatory response in the fetal membranes. Given the strong correlation between chorioamnionitis due to any agent and adverse pregnancy outcome, further studies to assess the effects of genital mycoplasmas on pregnancy outcome should be given high priority. It is worth bearing in mind that we (37) and others (116-118) have failed to isolated mycoplasmas from individuals with clear amniotic fluids at the time of amniocentesis. It is not known whether intra-amniotic hemmorrhage associated with discolored fluids predisposes to mycoplasmal infection or whether intra-amniotic infection caused the hemorrhage.

Peripartum Infection: M. hominis is the most common cause of postpartum fever (1-3,119) and is a cause of postpartum endometritis (120). Both M. hominis and U. urealyticum are a cause of postabortal fever (1-3). While these infections are often self-limited and do not require treatment, at least M. hominis septicemia results in a longer hospital stay and in some cases results in a suppurative septic arthritis (62-64) and post-cesarean wound infections (65).

Diseases of the Newborn: M. hominis is a cause of meningitis in the newborn (58) but the frequency with which it occurs is unknown. The features are similar to bacterial meningitis with low CSF glucose, elevated protein and a predominance of polymorphonuclear leukocytes. M. hominis is also a cause of septicemia (122), pericardial effusion (121), adenitis (59), and subcutaneous abscesses associated with breaks in the skin due to fetal monitoring electrodes (123) or forceps wounds (60).

Extragenital Infections in Adults: Extragenital infections in adults outside the peripartum period are being reported with increasing frequency. Self-limited M. hominis septicemia may occur in males with urinary tract abnormalities or manipulation (66). Wound infections due to M. hominis have occurred after mandibular fractures (68). Mandibular osteomyelitis developed in one of these cases and required tetracycline, sequestrectomy and removal of wire before healing. Brain abscesses (73) and a number of cases of septicemia (67,74,75) have been reported due to M. hominis. Other reports of extragenital M. hominis infections in adults mostly involve immunocompromised patients. A patient with a lymphoma on chemotherapy developed M. hominis septic arthritis following urinary tract instrumentation (69). Multiple sites of infection were found in two leukemic patients (70,71). A renal transplant recipient developed peritonitis and a wound infection from which M. hominis was isolated (72). The true incidence of extragenital infections due to either ureaplasmas or M. hominis is not known since these organisms are not routinely sought. Most of the reported cases have been discovered by "accident" due to the occasional growth of M. hominis blood agar (124) and in routine blood cultures (125).

SPECIFIC DISEASES FOR WHICH THERE IS STRONG, BUT NOT DEFINITIVE, EVIDENCE FOR A ROLE OF GENITAL MYCOPLASMAS

Urinary Tract: Although M. hominis plays an etiologic role in some cases of pyelonephritis, few convincing data ascribing a pathogenic role to this organism in lower urinary tract infections in women have been published. In contrast, present evidence suggests that U. urealyticum is a cause of the acute urethral syndrome (AUS) in women (20,21). In a recent study (20), counts of this organism of $> 10^3$/ml was associated with pyuria in women whose AUS had no other apparent etiology (the potential role of chlamydiae and other fastidious organisms were excluded) and the organism was isolated from suprapubic aspirates from four of 15 women with AUS of unknown etiology. Unfortunately, the isolation rate from bladder aspirated urine of control subjects was not determined. In an earlier study (19) by the same investigators where controls were examined, there was no difference in the isolation rate of ureaplasmas. However, urine from study patients collected by suprapubic aspiration was compared to midstream urine of controls.

The question of whether the high isolation rate from the lower genitourinary tract results in contamination of midstream urine and possible contamination of urine samples collected by suprapubic aspiration has not been evaluated. To circumvent these problems, we evaluated urine collected by open ended catheters from symptomatic patients with AUS of unknown etiology and asymptomatic patients matched for cervicovaginal colonization by ureaplasmas (21). Other infectious agents, including chlamydiae, were rigorously sought and those with polymicrobial infections were excluded. Not only were ureaplasmas isolated significantly more often from the urine of 17 symptomatic patients (89%) than from 37 control females (40%) but 65% of the symptomatic females had $>10^2$ ureaplasmas per ml of uncentrifuged urine versus 16% of the controls. The presence of $>10^2$/ml in symptomatic patients was associated with pyuria. Symptomatic women were culturally negative in the cervix/vagina and urethra for C. trachomatis. Evaluation of acute and convalescent serum from these patients by immunofluorescence indicated no recent exposure to C. trachomatis.

In another study of males and females (126), bladder-aspirate urine samples were cultured for the presence of fastidious microorganisms. These samples were obtained from 190 patients with urinary tract disease of symptoms suggesting infection of the urinary tract in whom standard bacteriologic investigation had failed to indicate bacterial infection. U. urealyticum was recovered alone or in association with other microorganisms from the bladder urine of 75% of patients with reflux scarring and abnormal renal function. Ureaplasmas were localized to the upper urinary tract in 80% of patients with bladder counts greater than $10^3$ colony-forming units per ml. Ureaplasmas were isolated from bladder urine of only 3% of control subjects.

There are several possible explanations for results obtained to date. *U. urealyticum* may be a normal inhabitant of the urinary bladder in healthy individuals and has no pathologic significance. However, the marked difference in the numbers of organisms present in patients versus control subjects suggests this is unlikely. A second possible explanation is that ureaplasmas are capable of colonizing previously damaged urinary tracts of individuals with diminished host resistance, but that such colonization is without pathologic significance. Finally, it is possible that ureaplasmas may infect normal or comprised urinary tracts and may cause or contribute to progressive disease.

*Genital Tract Disease:* A number of studies suggest that the prostate can be infected during the course of a ureaplasmal infection of the urethra (1-3). The most convincing data, however, are those from quantitative localization studies (17,18,127). In 82 (13.7%) of 597 patients with chronic prostatitis, a typical prostatitis histogram was observed for *U. urealyticum* (17). Eighty of these patients had high numbers of ureaplasmas in expressed prostatic secretions and 51 also in the first-voided urine after massage but in low or no numbers in first-voided or midstream urine. Although other fastidious organisms, including chlamydiae, were rigorously sought, only seven patients with ureaplasmal infection had other bacteria isolated from prostatic secretions. From 48 healthy persons, *U. urealyticum* was isolated from first voided urine from six and from none of midstream urines and from the expressed prostatic secretions of only one man and from none of the first-voided urines after massage. Seventy-one of the symptomatic patients were cured 21 to 28 days after treatment with tetracycline and ureaplasmas were no longer detected. Seven of the remaining eleven men had bladder neck obstruction. In four men, no obvious explanation for the therapy failure could be found. While it is difficult to determine whether organisms in prostatic secretions actually come from the prostate, it should be noted that other investigators (128) have isolated ureaplasmas from tissues obtained by perineal biopsy. While available evidence does not definitively prove a causal role for *U. urealyticum* in chronic prostatitis, they certainly suggest these organisms cannot be ignored as potential primary or contributory pathogens. Most studies have not found *M. hominis* to be associated with prostatitis. This is not too surprising in that urethritis often precedes prostatitis. *U. urealyticum* but not *M. hominis* is a cause of urethritis.

*Disorders of Reproductions: Infertility*. Given that *M. hominis* is a cause of salpingitis, it is reasonable to assume that severe tubal infection with this organism may lead to occlusion and infertility. However, prospective studies are needed to prove this.

Historically, infertility was one of the first conditions in humans in which ureaplasmas were suggested to play a role (2,3). Over 20 years later this association is still speculative. Over 50 articles purporting to prove or disprove the role of ureaplasmas in human infertility have been published in the last 10 years (35). Most studies have used one of two approaches: comparative isolation rates from the lower genital tracts of fertile and infertile couples and evidence of conception following antibiotic therapy. In general, these studies have suffered from one or more of the following defects: (i) failure to exclude possible involvement of other infectious agents, particularly chlamydiae, (ii) failure to include placebo treated controls, (iii) inadequate numbers of patients and controls so that statistical reliability is never achieved, (iv) failure to match the two groups for factors known to influence ureaplasmal colonization, (v) inadequate diagnostic evaluations of the patients, and (vi) limitation of investigation to epidemiological studies, which alone can suggest a relationship between ureaplasmas and disease, but never prove a cause and effect association. Furthermore, infertility is a syndrome, not a specific entity. Failure to incorporate this concept into experimental designs coupled with the high prevalence of the organism almost guarantees negative results. Only in two studies has the probability that ureaplasmas are likely to be related to infertility only in certain clinicopathological subsets been considered (35,129).

The most convincing evidence that ureaplasmas may be involved in infertility is that related to male factor(s). If in fact U. urealyticum is a cause of urethroprostatitis in some individuals and if prostatitis due to any agent is a cause of infertility, then one might reasonably suspect that ureaplasmas are a cause of male factor infertility. In a study of 194 infertile couples, one clinicopathological entity was identified, infertility associated with "male factor" (either alone or in conjunction with other causes of infertility), in which the incidence of U. urealyticum infection of the female's lower genital tract was over twice as high ($p < 0.005$) as in other infertile women (35). There were no statistically significant differences in the demographic data of this subpopulation as compared to the population of infertile women as a whole. In a similar study, other investigators (129) showed no correlation between ureaplasmal colonization and infertility, whether due to "male" or other factors. However, these investigators did not consider patients with multiple diagnoses in their analysis. This raises the possibility that ureaplasmal infection only plays a role in individuals subfertile for other reasons.

Other approaches to examining a causal role for U. urealyticum in male-related infertility have included the effect of ureaplasmas on semen quality, post-coital test, and antibiotic treatment. Results have been contradictory (1-3,35). However, in most cases, the effects of ureaplasmas were examined using infected and noninfected fertile individuals or infertile individuals with no controls.

Very few studies have been designed to investigate possible mechanisms whereby ureaplasmas may actually interfere with fertilization. There is one report of serotype differences in the ability of ureaplasmas to decrease the penetrating capacity of spermatozoa into zona-free hamster eggs (130). The deficiency in in vitro penetrating ability occurred only when sperm were incubated with serotypes 4,6, and 8. Pretreatment of eggs with ureaplasmas did not significantly alter penetration.

To definitively prove whether or not U. urealyticum is involved in human infertility will require different experimental approaches than most of those that have been used. Additional studies comparing isolation rates between unselected populations of fertile and infertile individuals are unlikely to provide any useful data. Instead future epidemiological studies should concentrate on well-defined clinicopathological studies and isolation rates should be determined both for lower and upper tracts. Methods in obtaining cultural specimens from the upper tract should be ones documented to preclude cervical contamination. Studies where this has been taken into account indicate that both M. hominis and U. urealyticum can be isolated from the endometrium of infertile individuals in the absence of other bacteria, chlamydiae, and viruses (35). M. hominis was isolated from the endometrium of 2 of 33 individuals infected with this organism in the vagina/cervix and U. urealyticum from 1 of 77 individuals infected in the lower genital tract. Additional studies involving larger number of patients should be undertaken to determine the potential significance of these findings.

If subpopulations are identified in which U. urealyticum may play a role, careful in vitro and in vivo studies need to be conducted to identify possible pathogenic mechanisms. The later is likely to require animal models for definitive results. Precaution should be taken to select a species and strain of animal which is susceptible to ureaplasmal infection and that multiple reference serotypes are utilized for inoculation as well as multiple clinical isolates. Different animal species differ in their susceptibility to ureaplasmal induced urethritis (131) and/or different ureaplasmal strains (132). Most importantly, only animals documented to be free of mycoplasmas and other pathogenic organisms should be used.

Currently, there is sufficient reason to justify intensive efforts only in male factor infertility. Additional studies in this area need to obtain quantitative cultural data, and imply more quantitative assays to measure semen parameters. Studies to examine the effects of U. urealyticum upon interactions of spermatozoa with human ova, are particularly likely to prove enlightening. In all of these possibilities, semen from infected individuals with male factor infertility should be compared to that from infected fertile individuals and that from infected infertile individuals.

Pregnancy Outcome: Present evidence indicates that both U. urealyticum and M. hominis can cause a clinically silent infection of the endometrium (35) and can invade the amnionic sac as early as the sixteenth week of gestation, even in the presence of a viable, apparently healthy fetus and intact fetal membranes (37). Importantly, U. urealyticum can cause a slowly progressing, clinically silent amniotic fluid infection (37). That these organisms do so at a rather high frequency is suggested by their isolation from the endometrium of 20% of unselected individuals with intact fetal membranes at the time of cesarean section (133) and from the placentas of 11% of unselected individuals with intact membranes and no labor undergoing cesarean section (109). These facts taken in conjunction with the striking association of ureaplasmal infection of the placenta and chorioamnionitis (38-40) at the time of delivery strongly suggest that these organisms may be a major cause of adverse pregnancy outcome. While epidemiological studies to date are not definitive, those based upon placental, not lower genital tract, are supportive of a role of ureaplasmas in prematurity and low birth weight and perinatal morbidity and mortality (38-40). They are suggestive of a role in habitual spontaneous abortion.

Spontaneous abortion: U. urealyticum and M. hominis have been implicated in spontaneous abortion, in some cases in association with maternal septicemia (1-3). The organisms have been isolated from fetal lungs, brain, heart and viscera (1-3,134). U. urealyticum has been isolated more frequently from the products of early abortions and mid-trimester fetal losses than from products of induced abortions (134,135). Although rates of isolation of ureaplasmas from the lower genital tract of habitual aborters do not differ from normal controls, ureaplasmas are isolated more often from the endometrium of habitual aborters (136). U. urealyticum but not M. hominis is isolated more frequently from the placentas of aborted fetuses than from controls (38,40). Antibody titers to U. urealyticum are higher in mothers with a history of fetal wastage (137). Complement-fixing antibody to M. hominis has been found more commonly after abortion than in normal pregnant women

(138) whereas the occurrence of the organism in the cervix of the two groups of women was not different. However, increase in antibody titer to *M. hominis* occurs in some women during or after a normal pregnancy (139). Unfortunately, the results of all of these epidemiological studies are difficult to interpret since the comparability of the various groups of women is uncertain and the role of other microorganisms was often not assessed. While the placental studies took this into account, they did not take into account the duration of labor. Several studies have indicated an increase in the number of normal pregnancies following treatment with broadspectrum antibiotics or erythromycin (140,141) but these trials either been uncontrolled or the numbers of patients too few.

*Prematurity and Low Birth Weight*: The first suggestion that infection might be involved in prematurity and low birth weight resulted from studies where tetracycline was administered to nonbacteriuric, pregnant women on a double-blind basis (143). Women who were treated for 6 weeks during pregnancy gave birth to significantly fewer infants weighting 2500g or less than women given a placebo. Although no microbiological investigations were conducted, it was postulated that tetracycline-sensitive microorganisms might be responsible, and mycoplasmas were considered among these. More recently, a study was performed in which pregnant women whose cultures were positive for either *U. urealyticum*, *M. hominis* or both, were given, in a double blind protocol, either erythromycin (active against *U. urealyticum*), clindamycin (active against *M. hominis*) or a placebo (44). The effect of erythromycin treatment in lowering rates of low birth weight was substantial. Presumably much of the effect of the erythromycin was anti-ureaplasmal, but an effect on other infectious agents is possible. In the study population, the rate of carriage of *C. trachomatis* was approximately 4-6%; therefore, it is unlikely that the effect of erythromycin is completely explained by an anti-chlamydial action. It was felt unlikely that anaerobes accounted for the effect of erythromycin, in that clindamycin did not seem to have as striking an effect.

Only one prospective study based upon isolation of *U. urealyticum* and *M. hominis* from the cervix has shown an association with low birth weight. In this study by Braun, *et al*. (13), women who were colonized with *U. urealyticum* delivered babies whose mean birth weight was 202g less than that of babies of uninfected women (p .003). *M. hominis*, often co-isolated with *U. urealyticum*, was less well-linked with low birth weight (p=.054). This study involved women of low income, greater than 60% of whom were black. When stratified by ethnic group, the only significant association was that of *U. urealyticum* with low birth weight infants of black women. Interestingly, none of four other studies (45-48) trying to repeat this work evaluated a significant number of blacks; none showed an effect. In fact, one was limited strictly to women of upper income (48), two (46,47) evaluated insufficient numbers of patients (199 and 104 patients); the remaining study (45) was well controlled but only 3.5% were black. Whether the strong association between the presence of *U. urealyticum* in black mothers and low birth weight represents an etiologic relationship or merely identifies patients with an underlying predisposition toward babies of low birth weight cannot be determined. It can be said with certainty, however, that blacks are more likely to be infected with ureaplasmas than whites even when sexual experience is taken into account (2). A recent study based on vaginal isolation in a predominantly black, lower socioeconomic patient population, failed to find a association of ureaplasmal infection with low birth weight but did find an association with preterm labor (143).

In the study by Braun, et al., (13) 84% of pregnant women had mycoplasmas in the urogenital tract, 79% with U. urealyticum and 48% with M. hominis (many were coinfected). Only 8.5% of babies weighed less than 2500g; therefore, it is apparent that factors other than the mere presence of mycoplasmas are of importance in influencing birth weight. One possibility is invasion of the upper genital tract by mycoplasmas. In fact, others have shown in the same patient population as Braun and coworkers, that rises in antibody titers to U. urealyticum, but not M. hominis, delineate a group of pregnancies with two to three-fold higher risks of low-birth-weight delivery (44). Infants born to women with antibody rises were distributed among the various categories of low birth weight and prematurity. There were about equal numbers in the groups with shortened gestational age, and the small-for-gestational-age group, thus indicating that the effect of U. urealyticum on outcome of pregnancy is not limited to any one subcategory.

Two studies (12,55) based upon isolation of U. urealyticum from the nose and throat (but not genital tract) of infants have shown a strong association with infant colonization and low birth weight. M. hominis colonization was also found to be associated but to a lesser degree. In view of the high frequency of occurrence of M. hominis with U. urealyticum, the association found between M. hominis and birth weight may reflect only the effect of U. urealyticum. Neither organism was linked to shortened gestation nor to such known risk factors for low birth weight as previous history of prematurity, abortion, stillbirth, cigarette smoking, bacteriuria, or development of toxemia or third trimester hemmorrhage (12). However, the groups were small and as recently emphasized by Harrison, et al. (45) the data are open to question because multivariate analysis techniques were not utilized.

Three studies have examined the relationship between colonization of the placenta and low birth weight. Two showed an association (38,39). Naessens et al. (48) cultured placentas for U. urealyticum but not M. hominis from 253 women, all of upper income. There was no significant difference in the birth weight of infants whose placentas were colonized.

Embree, et al. (38) cultured placentas from a group of 446 "high-risk" pregnancies and 108 unselected deliveries of normal full term infants. Isolation of U. urealyticum, but not M. hominis, was associated with prematurity, lower birth weight, and intrauterine growth retardation (IUGR). As the gestational age or birth weight of the infants increased, the isolation rate of U. urealyticum decreased. U. urealyticum was isolated from 32% of the placentas from infants under 38 weeks gestation, significantly more often ($p < .001$) than from the control infants of greater than 37 weeks gestation (9%). Except for spontaneous abortions, M. hominis was isolated only from placentas of infants over 31 weeks gestation. U. urealyticum was isolated from 34% of placentas of infants weighing less than 2500g in the high risk group. This was significantly greater ($p < .001$) than the isolation rate of 9% of placentas in the control group, in which the infants' birth weights were all greater than 2500. In the high risk group, birth weights of infants over 38 weeks gestation from whom U. urealyticum was isolated from the placenta averaged 3218; the difference, 308g, between their average weight and that of controls was also statistically significant ($p < .001$). The association between U. urealyticum colonization and low birth weight was not influenced by maternal smoking, toxemia, or gestational diabetes.

Knudsin, et al. (39) evaluated the presence of ureaplasmas, mycoplasmas, chlamydiae, fungi, aerobic and anaerobic bacteria, and cytomegalovirus in fetal membranes and evaluated their association with perinatal morbidity and mortality. They cultured 801 placentas from three groups of subjects (144 who died in the perinatal period, 452 neonates admitted to the intensive-care unit, and 205 case matched controls). U. urealyticum, M. hominis, or both were isolated from 21% of placentas of premature and term infants who died in the perinatal period, 25% of those admitted to intensive care, and 11% of controls. Gestational age and birth weight were inversely related to isolation of U. urealyticum. Among intensive-care infants, the percentage of positive placental cultures declined progressively, from a rate of 39% in infants under 1000g to 16% in infants of 2500g or more. Among placentas associated with perinatal deaths, the isolation rate of ureaplasmas, was also highest in infants with the lowest birth weights. Among all subjects, recovery of ureaplasmas from the placenta showed a strong inverse relationship to birth weight. Similar results were obtained when data were analyzed according to gestational age. When superimposed on the standard intrauterine-weight chart of Lubchenco et al. (144), all data fell in the range of the 50th percentile, indicating an appropriate relationship between birth weight and gestational age in both ureaplasma-positive and negative subjects. With respect to the strong association between U. urealyticum colonization and low birth weight, these investigators assessed possible confounding with maternal characteristics including spontaneous rupture of membranes, preeclampsia, maternal age less than 25 yr, primagravidity, marital status, race, occupation, diabetes, and smoking. Three of these were significantly associated with low birth weight; colonization with U. urealyticum, spontaneous rupture of membranes, and preeclampsia. With regard to the association with preeclampsia, it is of interest that U. urealyticum is isolated more frequently (rate 20%), and usually in higher numbers, from bladder aspirated urine of patients with preeclampsia than from that of healthy pregnant pregnant women (rate, 7%) (23).

In summary, the association of U. urealyticum with low birth weight remains controversial. Available evidence suggests that maternal cervical colonization is not consistently correlated with low birth weight. In contrast, colonization of the placenta in "high risk" pregnancies with U. urealyticum is strongly associated. This suggests that only a subpopulation of those women infected in the cervix are at risk for delivering low birth weight infants. While studies of placentas have taken into account the time of membrane rupture, they have not considered the duration of labor nor the presence and numbers of U. urealyticum in the cervix/vagina of study and control patients. Future studies should not only take this into account but should also determine the presence of chorioamnionitis and the possible presence of a broad range of genital pathogens. In a prospective study in which a comprehensive attempt was made to detect microorganisms of all types in 57 amniotic fluids collected at sixteen to twenty weeks of gestation, U. urealyticum was isolated in pure culture from two and M. hominis in pure culture from two (37). Both of the individuals from whom U. urealyticum was isolated and one of the individuals from whom M. hominis was isolated had premature labor and rupture of the membranes. The former at six and seven weeks following amniocentesis with both resulting in early neonatal death and isolation of ureaplasmas in pure culture from the placenta of both and fetal tissues in one. Severe choreioamnionitis was present in both placentas from which ureaplasmas were isolated and mild inflammation was present in one of the two from which M. hominis was isolated. Thus it seems that in some instances, U. urealyticum may cause premature rupture of the membranes. Since 70-80% of all perinatal deaths not attributable to congenital malformations occur in neonates born prematurely (145), further investigation of the causal role of U. urealyticum in prematurity should be given high priority.

Perinatal Morbidity and Mortality: Based upon well documented case reports, there is no question that both U. urealyticum (37,131,132,158) and M. hominis (42,43) can cause perinatal morbidity and mortality (37,41,49-53,121). Recent prospective studies suggest that ureaplasmas in particular may be a common cause (38-40). In a recent study of 33 perinatal deaths (28 stillborn and 5 who died within 48 hours of birth) and 31 random cases of normal term deliveries, genital mycoplasmas were said to have been isolated significantly more often from cases in which death of the fetus could not be attributed to a known anatomic or morphologic cause than from controls (40). Also, the lungs and placentas were more likely to be inflamed in positive study cases than in controls. Antibody titers to genital mycoplasmas were also more likely to be elevated in these mothers and neonates. Unfortunately, interpretation is made difficult because the data for ureaplasmas and M. hominis in this study were not always analyzed separately. Also in many cases of analysis, a case was considered positive if it was serologically positive even though it was culture negative. If only culture proven cases are considered and the cases from which other pathogenic organisms were coisolated are excluded, then it is not clear whether the results would remain statistically significant. Interpretation of the data are further complicated because the duration of labor was not taken into account, and the study and control infants were not matched for gestational age. In another study (39) in which all of these aspects were considered, except duration of labor, U. uealyticum, M. hominis, or both were still isolated more frequently from the placentas of premature and term infants who died in the perinatal period and from the placentas from those neonates admitted to the intensive-care unit than from case matched controls.

Respiratory disease is the most common cause of perinatal morbidity and mortality, especially in premature infants (146). There is some evidence to suggest that congenital pneumonia or pneumonia acquired during birth is almost always accompanied by chorioamnionitis (147). As already discussed, the one infectious agent most commonly associated with chorioamnionitis and prematurity is U. urealyticum. Retrospective studies indicate an association of U. urealyticum and M. hominis with congenital pneumonia (149). Both have been isolated directly from fetal lung tissue (37,41,49-53). U. urealyticum has been isolated from affected lungs in the absence of bacteria, fungi, viruses, and chlamydiae (37,49), and has been demonstrated within lung lesions by electron and immunofluorescent microscopy (49). This organism can induce ciliostasis and mucosal lesions in human fetal tracheal organ cultures (49). Quinn, et al. (54) showed a significant association between a metabolism inhibition (MI) antibody response to U. urealyticum and respiratory distress in newborn infants. Unfortunately, the controls in these studies were term infants and were not appropriately matched for factors predictive of ureaplasmal colonization; thus they were not comparable. Furthermore, because infants with respiratory distress receive almost daily blood transfusions, serology must be interpreted with great caution, especially in the absence of cultural data as was done in this study. Also, results should be evaluated on the basis of antibody levels in donor serum not that of the mother, as was done in this study. Even though packed cells are administered in the transfusions, these contain a minimum of 20% donor plasma (149).

Two recent studies have been unable to demonstrate a relationship between isolation of U. urealyticum from the newborn infant and respiratory disease. In a prospective study carried out by Rudd, et al. (55) in London, nasopharyngeal aspirates were taken from 235 newborn infants admitted to the neonatal intensive care unit. U. urealyticum was isolated from 53/235 (22%). Isolation was significantly associated with preterm birth, low birth weight, and membranes ruptured for more than 24 hours prior to delivery. Colonization of the respiratory tract was present in 16/41 (39%) of infants of 28 weeks gestation or less, but in only 3/30 (10%) of babies at term. Although the organisms were isolated more commonly in babies with respiratory distress, those requiring prolonged oxygen treatment, or apnea, when the effect of gestation was considered, these relationships were not significant. Of course, if ureaplasmas are a cause of shortened gestation, then separation of the two might be impossible.

An enzyme-linked immunosorbent assay (ELISA) was used in a randomly selected sample of infants from the study of Rudd, et al. (150) to evaluate the serological response to U. urealyticum. The ELISA tested for all known serotypes of ureaplasmas and the assay has a sensitivity comparable to that of the metabolic inhibition (MI) test (96). Those analyzing the samples had no knowledge of the isolation results. U. urealyticum specific IgG was found in 6/41 babies tested. Of the 41 infants, 23 were colonized with U. urealyticum, and this organism was isolated from all 6 babies where antibody was present. Specimens were analyzed from 16 babies who were colonized with U. urealyticum and had prolonged periods of oxygen treatment but neither IgM or IgA were detected. It is of interest that M. hominis specific IgA and IgM were detected in a number of infants with pneumonia.

In another study from England, Taylor-Robinson et al. (56) obtained throat swabs or gastric aspirates from 47 infants with respiratory disease, and 49 controls of similar gestational age. U. urealyticum was isolated from 29% of infants delivered vaginally but there was no evidence that the organism contributed to respiratory disease.

Gallo et al. (57) showed an antibody response to U. urealyticum may occur in infants but is unusual. Serum specimens were collected from 713 newborns with suspected viral and chlamydial infections (Gallo personal communication) during the neonatal period and infancy; and measurement of IgG and IgM antibodies was performed using an indirect immunofluorescent test. In 17 babies (2.4%) IgM antibody was detected. Of the 10 infants with symptoms from birth in whom IgM antibody was detected, none had pneumonia. Six of the other 7 babies had respiratory infections with onset between 3-13 weeks after birth; there was serological evidence of rubella infection in one and C. trachomatis infection in two infants.

In a study performed at the University of Alabama at Birmingham, infants aged 2-12 weeks with pneumonitis were evaluated for disease due to the more fastidious infectious agents (151). Infants with bronchopulmonary dysplasia and those with acute lobar pneumonia were excluded. The isolation rate from nasopharyngeal aspirates of these infants was compared to that of hospitalized, age-matched controls. Although the cervicovaginal isolation rate did not differ between mother of study infants and controls, U. urealyticum was isolated significantly more often from the nasophryngeal aspirates of infants with pneumonitis [8/38 (21%)] than from controls [2/49 (4%)]. Of the 8 isolates of U. urealyticum, 6 were associated with other organisms; cytomegalovirus 3, Pneumocystis carinii 3, C. trachomatis 2, and Bordetella pertussis 1. Thus it would seem that at least in most cases U. urealyticum is a secondary, not a primary pathogen of the respiratory tract.

The apparent discrepancy between the striking association between chorioamnionitis and U. urealyticum and its apparent lack of association with respiratory disease is difficult to reconcile. However, neither of the two prospective cultural studies were based upon isolation of the organism directly from affected lung, i.e. tracheal aspirates. Culture of the nasopharynx and/or gastric aspirates is not reliable for diagnosis of lower respiratory tract disease (152). Unfortunately, culture of tracheal aspirates even using the best of methods may result in erroneous information due to contamination of sample with upper respiratory tract secretions. A prospective study based upon culture of blood and cerebrospinal fluid as well as tracheal aspirates and IgM specific responses in blood collected prior to transfusion should be more meaningful. Ultimately, therapy trials may best provide the evidence of the causal role.

SUMMARY

U. urealyticum and M. hominis can no longer be considered as harmless commensals of the lower genitourinary tract. Both can produce disease in humans. Diagnosis and management of infections due to these organisms must be based upon isolation of the organisms from the affected site and preferably the number of organisms present. Due to the frequent resistance of both organisms to tetracycline (153,154), treatment must be based upon appropriate antibiotic sensitivities. For a more detailed description of the basic biology of these organisms and isolation and identification and treatment, the reader is referred to several recent reviews (1-3).

REFERENCES

1. Taylor-Robinson, D. and W.M. McCormack, The genital mycoplasmas. N. Engl. J. Med. 302:1003,1063, 1980.
2. McCormack, W.M. and D. Taylor-Robinson, The genital mycoplasmas in sexually transmitted diseases. K.K. Holmes, P.A. Mardh, P.F. Sparling, and P.J. Wiesner, Eds., McGraw-Hill Company, New York, pp. 408-419, 1984.
3. Cassell, G.H. and B.C. Cole, Mycoplasmas as agents of human disease. N. Engl. J. Med. 304:80, 1981.
4. Tully, J.G., D. Taylor-Robinson, R.M. Cole, et al., A newly discovered mycoplasma in the human urogenital tract. Lancet 1:1288, 1981.
5. Taylor-Robinson, D., J.G. Tully, P.M. Furr, et al,. Urogenital mycoplasma infection of man: a review with observations on a recently discovered mycoplasma. Isr. J. Med. Sci. 17:524, 1981.
6. Tully, J.G., D. Taylor-Robinson, D.L. Rose, et al., Mycoplasma genitalium, a new species from the human urogenital tract. Int. J. Syst. Bacteriol 33:387, 1983.
7. Moller, B.R., D. Taylor-Robinson and P.M. Furr, Serological evidence implicating Mycoplasma genitalium in pelvic inflammatory disease. Lancet i:1102, 1984.
8. Taylor-Robinson, D., P.M. Furr and C.M. Hetherington, The pathogenicity of a newly discovered human mycoplasma (strain G37) for the genital tract of marmosets. J. Hyg. 89:449, 1982.
9. Moller, B.R., D. Taylor-Robinson, P.M. Furr, et al, Acute upper genital-tract disease in female monkeys provoked experimentally by Mycoplasma genitalium. Brit. J. Exp. Pathol. 66:417, 1985.
10. Taylor-Robinson, D., J.G. Tully and M.F. Barile, Urethral infection in male chimpanzees produced experimentally by Mycoplasma genitalium. Brit. J. Exp. Pathol. 66:95, 1985.
11. McCormack, W.M. Epidemiology of Mycoplasma hominis. Sex. Trans. Dis. 4(suppl):261, 1983.
12. Klein, J.O., D. Buckland and M. Finland, Colonization of newborn infants by mycoplasmas. N. Engl. J. Med. 280:1025, 1969.
13. Braun, P., Y-H Lee, J.O. Klein et al., Birth weight and genital mycoplasmas in pregnancy. N.J. Engl. Med. 284:167, 1971.
14. Foy, H.M., G.E. Kenny and E.M. Levinsohn, Acquisition of

mycoplasmata and T strains during infancy. J. Infect. Dis. 121:579, 1970.

15. Taylor-Robinson, D. Ureaplasmas as a cause of disease in man and animals: Fact or fancy? Isr. J. Med. Sci. 20:843, 1984.
16. Taylor-Robinson, D, G.W. Csonka and M.J. Prentice, Human intraurethral inoculation of ureaplasmas. Quart. J. Med. 46:309, 1977.
17. Brunner, H., W. Weidner and H-GI Schiefer, Quantitative studies on the role of Ureaplasma urealyticum in non-gonococcal urethritis and chronic prostatitis. Yale J. Biol. Med. 56:545, 1983.
18. Brunner, H., W. Weidner and H-G Schiefer, Studies on the role of Ureaplasma urealyticum and Mycoplasma hominis in prostatitis. J. Infect. Dis. 147:807, 1983.
19. Stamm, W.E., K.F. Wagner, R. Amsel, et al., Causes of the acute urethral syndrome in women. N. Engl. J. Med. 303:409, 1980.
20. Stamm, W.E., K. Running, J. Hale, et al., Etiologic role of Mycoplasma hominis and Ureaplasma urealyticum in women with the acute urethral syndrome. Sex. Trans. Dis. 10 (suppl):319, 1983.
21. Brown, M.B., K.B. Waites, S. Stagno, et al., Association of Ureaplasma urealyticum with the Urethral Syndrome of Females: Demonstration by quantitative cutlure of urine collected by catheterization (submitted for publication).
22. Thomsen, A.C. Occurrence and pathogenicity of Mycoplasma hominis in the upper urinary tract: A review. Sex. Trans. Dis. 4(suppl):323, 1983.
23. Savige, J.A., G.L. Gilbert, K.F. Fairley, et al., Bacteriuria due to Ureaplasma urealyticum and Gardnerella vaginalis in women with preeclmapsia. J. Infect. Dis. 148:605, 1983.
24. Birch, D.F., A.J.F. D'Apice and K.F. Fairley, Ureaplasma urealyticum in the upper urinary tracts of renal allograft recipients. J. Infect. Dis. 144:123, 1981.
25. McDowall, D.R., J.D. Buchanan, K.F. Fairley, et al., Anaerobic and other fastidious microorganisms in asymptomatic bacteriuria in pregnant women. 144:114, 1981.
26. Mardh, P.A., L. Westrom and S. Colen, Infections of the genital and urinary tracts with mycoplasmas and ureaplasma. In genital infections and their complications. D. Danielsson, L. Juhlin and P.A. Mardh, eds. Almquist and Viskell, Stockholm, pp. 53, 1975.
27. Petterson, S., J.E. Broson, L. Grenabo, et al., Ureaplasma urealyticum in infectious urinary stones. Lancet 1:526, 1983.
28. Clerc, M., J. Texier and C. Babear, Experimental production of bladder calculi in rats by Ureaplasma injection. Ann. Microbiol. (Inst. Pasteur) 135A:135, 1984.
29. Friedlander, A.M. and A.I. Braude, Production of bladder stones by human T mycoplasmas. Nature (Lond.) 247:67, 1974.
30. Grenabo, L., J-E Broson, H. Hedelin, et al., Ureaplasma urealyticum-induced crystallization of magnesium ammonium phosphate and calcium phosphates in synthetic urine. J. Urol. 132:795.
31. Mardh, P.-A. and L. Westrom, Tubal and cervical cultures in acute salpingitis with special reference to Mycoplasma hominis and T-strain mycoplasmas. Br. J. Vener. Dis. 46:179, 1970.
32. Mardh, P.-A. Mycoplasmal PID: A review of natural and experimental infections. Yale J. Biol. Med. 56:529, 1983.
33. Miettinen, A., J. Paavonen, E. Jansson, et al., Enzyme immunoassay for serum antibody to Mycoplasma hominis in women with acute pelvic inflammatory disease. Sex. Trans. Dis. 10(suppl):289, 1983.
34. Henry-Suchet, J., F. Catalan, V. Loffredo, et al., Microbiology of specimens obtained by laparoscopy from controls and from patients with pelvic inflammatory disease or infertility with tuboal obstruction. Chlamydia trachomatis and Ureaplasma urealyticum, Am. J. Obstet. Gynecol. 138:1022, 1980.

35. Cassell, G.H., B.J. Younger, M.B. Brown, et al., Microbiologic study of infertile women at the time of diagnostic laparascopy: Association of Ureaplasma urealyticum with a defined subpopulation. N. Engl. J. Med. 308:502, 1983.
36. Capsi, E., E. Herczeg, F. Solomon, et al., Amnioitis and T strain mycoplasmemia. Am. J. Obstet. Gynecol. 111:1102, 1971.
37. Cassell, G.H., R.O. Davis, K.B. Waites, et al., Isolation of Mycoplasma hominis and Ureaplasma urealyticum from amniotic fluid at 16-20 weeks of gestation: Potential effect on outcome of pregnancy. Sex. Trans. Dis. 10(suppl):294, 1983.
38. Embree, J.E., V.W. Kraus, J.A. Embil, et al., Placental infection with Mycoplasma hominis and Ureaplasma urealyticum: Clinical correlation. Obstet. Gynecol. 56:475, 1980.
39. Kundsin, R.B., S.G. Driscoll and R.R. Monson, Association of Ureaplasma urealyticum in the placenta with perinatal morbidity and mortality. N. Engl. J. Med. 310:941, 1984.
40. Quinn, P.A., J. Butany, M. Chipman, et al., A prospective study of microbial infection in stillbirths and early neonatal death. Am. J. Obstet. Gynecol. 151:238, 1985.
41. Dische, R.M., P.A. Quinn, E. Czegledy-Nagy, et al., Genital mycoplasma infection. Intrauterine infection: Pathologic study of the fetus and placenta. Am. J. Clin. Pathol. 72:167, 1979.
42. Kundsin, R.B. and S.G. Driscoll, The role of mycoplasmas in human reproductive failure. Ann. N.Y. Acad. Sci. 174:794, 1970.
43. Harrison, R.H., E.R. Alexander, L. Weinstein, et al., Cervical Chlamydia trachomatis and mycoplasmal infections in pregnancy. J.A.M.A. 250:1721, 1983.
44. Kass, E.H., W.M. McCormack, J-S Lin, et al., Genital mycoplasmas as a cause of excess premature delivery. Trans. Assoc. Am. Physicians. 94:261, 1981.
45. Harrison, R.F., R. Hurley and J. de Louvois, Genital mycoplasmas and birth weight in offspring of primigravid women. Am. J. Obstet. Gynecol. 133:201, 1979.
46. Ross, J.M., P.M. Furr, D. Taylor-Robinson, et al., The effect of genital mycoplasmas on human fetal growth. Br. J. Obstet. Gynecol. 88:749, 1981.
47. Foy, H.M., G.E. Kenny, W.L. Wentworth, et al., Isolation of Mycoplasma hominis T-strains and cytomegalovirus from the cervix of pregnant women. Am. J. Obstet. Gynecol. 106:635, 1970.
48. Naessens, A., W. Foulon, M. Volkckaert, et al., Cervical and placental colonization by Ureaplasma urealyticum in pregnant women and fetal outcome. J. Infect. Dis. 148:333, 1983.
49. Quinn, P.A., J.E. Gilan, T. Markstad, et al., Intrauterine infection with Ureaplasma urealyticum as a cause of fatal neonatal pneumonia. Pediatr. Infect. Dis. 4:538, 1985.
50. Tafari, N., S. Ross, R.L. Naeye, et al., Mycoplasma T strains and perinatal death. Lancet 1:108, 1976.
51. Romano, N., F. Romano and F. Carollo, T-strains of mycoplasmas in broncopneumonic lungs of an aborted fetus. N. Engl. J. Med. 285:950, 1971.
52. Brunnell, P.A., M.R. Dische and M. Walker, Mycoplasma amnionitis and respiratory distress syndrome. J.A.M.A. 207:2097, 1969.
53. Pease, P., K.B. Rogers and B.C. Cole, A cytopathogenic strain of Mycoplasma hominis type 1 isolated from the lung of a stillborn infant. J. Pathol. Bacteriol. 94:460, 1967.
54. Quinn, P.A., S. Rubin, D.M. Nocilla, et al., Serologic evidence of Ureaplasma urealyticum infection in neonatal respiratory disease. Yale J. Biol. Med. 56:565, 1983.
55. Rudd, P.T. and D. Carrington, A prospective study of chlamydial mycoplasmal and viral infections in a neonatal intensive care unit. Arch. Dis. Child. 59:120, 1984.

56. Taylor-Robinson, D., P.M. Furr and M.M. Liberman, The occurrence of genital mycoplasmas in babies with and without respiratory disease. Acta. Pediatr. Scand. 73:383, 1984.
57. Gallo, D., K.W. Dupuis, N.J. Schmidt, et al., Broadly reactive immunofluorescence test for measurement of immunoglobulin M and G antibodies to Ureaplasma urealyticum in infant and adult sera. J. Clin. Microbiol. 17:614.
58. Mardh, P.A. Mycoplasma hominis infection of the central nervous system in newborn infants. Sex. Trans. Dis. 10(suppl):331, 1983.
59. Powell, D.A., K. Miller and W.A. Clyde, Submandibular adenitis in a newborn infant caused by Mycoplasma hominis. Pediatrics. 63:798, 1979.
60. Sacker, I., M. Walker and P.A. Brunell, Abscess in newborn infant caused by Mycoplasma. Pediatrics 46:303, 1970.
61. Gewitz, M., R. Dinwiddie, L. Rees, et al., Mycoplasma hominis. A cause of neonatal meningitis. Arch. Dis. Child. 54:231, 1979.
62. Verninder, D.G.R. Septic arthritis due to Mycoplasma hominis. J. Bone Joint Surg. 60:224, 1978.
63. Anonymous, Mycoplasma hominis infection. Br. Med. J. 2:766, 1976.
64. Anonymous, Mycoplasma hominis infection. Br. Med. J. 3:816, 1974.
65. Solomon, F., E. Caspi, I. Bukovsky and D. Sompolinsky. Infections associated with genital mycoplasmas. Am. J. Obstet Gynecol. 116:785, 1973.
66. Simberkoff, M.S. and B. Toharsky, Mycoplasmemia in adult male patients. J.A.M.A. 236:2522, 1976.
67. Ti, Ty, M. Dan, G.W. Stemke, J.A. Robertson and G. Goldsand, Isolation of Mycoplasma hominis from the blood of men with multiple trauma and fever. J.A.M.A. 247:60, 1982.
68. Lee, Y., R.R. Nersasian, N.K. Lan, A. McDonald and W.M. McCormack, Wound infections with Mycoplasma hominis. J.A.M.A. 218:252, 1971.
69. McDonald, M.K., J.O. Moore, J.M. Harrelson, C.P. Browning and H.A. Gallis, Septic arthritis due to Mycoplasma hominis, Arth. Rheum. 26:1044, 1983.
70. DeGirolami, P.C. and S. Madoff, Mycoplasma hominis septicemia. J. Clin. Micro. 16:566, 1982.
71. Friis, H, A. Plesner, J. Scheibel, T. Justesen and K. Lind, Mycoplasma hominis septicemia. Br. Med. J. 286:2103, 1983.
72. Mokhbat, J.E., P.K. Peterson and L.D. Sabath; Peritonitis due to Mycoplasma hominis in a renal transplant patient. J. Infect. Dis. 146:713, 1982.
73. Payan, D.G., N. Seigal and S. Madoff, Infection of a brain abscess by Mycoplasma hominis. 14:571, 1981.
74. Boe, O., O.E. Iversen, A. Mehl, Septicemia due to Mycoplasma hominis. Scand. J. Infect. Dis. 15:87, 1983.
75. Spencer, R.C. and C.B. Brown, Septicaemia in a renal transplant patient due to Mycoplasma hominis. 6:267, 1983.
76. Taylor-Robinson, D., B.J. Thomas, P.M. Furr, et al., The association of Mycoplasma hominis with arthritis. Sex. Trans. Dis. 10(suppl):341, 1983.
77. Stuckey, M., P.A. Quinn and E.W. Gelfand, Identification of Ureaplasma urealyticum (T-strain mycoplasma) in a patient with polyarthritis. Lancet 2:917, 1978.
78. Webster, A.D.B., D. Taylor-Robinson, P.M. Furr, et al., Mycoplasmal (ureaplasmal) septic arthritis in hypogammaglobulinaemia. Br. Med. J. 1:478, 1978.
79. Vogler, L.B., K.B. Waites, P.F. Wright, et al., Ureaplasma urealyticum polyarthritis in agammaglobulinemia. Pedistr. Infect. Dis. 4:687, 1985.
80. Doig, P.A., H.L. Ruhnke and N.C. Palmer, Experimental bovine genital ureaplasmosis. II. Granular vulvitis, endometritis, and salpingitis following uterine inoculation. Can. J. Comp. Med. 44:259, 1980.

81. Howard, C.J., R.N. Gourlay and J. Brownlie, Immunity in experimental T-mycoplasmal mastitis. Infect. Immun. 9:400, 1974.
82. Ruhnke, H.L., N.C. Palmer, P.A. Doig, et al., Bovine abortion and neonatal death associated with Ureaplasma diversum. Theriogenology 21:295.
83. Miller, R.B., H.L. Ruhnke, P.A. Doig, et al., The effects of Ureaplasma diversum inoculated into the amniotic cavity in cows. Theriogenology 20:367, 1983.
84. Howard, C.J., R.N. Gourlay, L.H. Thomas, et al., Induction of pneumonia in gnotobiotic calves following inocualtion of Mycoplasma dispar and ureaplasmas (T-mycoplasmas). Res. Vet. Sci. 21:227, 1976.
85. Moller, B.R., E.A. Freundt, F.T. Black, et al., Experimental infection of the genital tract of female grivet monkeys by Mycoplasma hominis. Infect. Immun. 20:248, 1978.
86. Mardh, P.A., L. Westrom and C. Mecklenburg, Studies on ciliated epithelia of the human genital tract. I. Swelling of the cilia of fallopian tube epithelium in organ cultures infected with Mycoplasma hominis. Brit. J. Vener. Dis. 52:52, 1976.
87. Moller, B.R., F.T. Black and E.A. Freundt, Attempts to produce gynaecological disease in grivet monkeys with Ureaplasma urealyticum. J. Med. Microbiol. 14:475, 1981.
88. Taylor-Robinson, D., and F.E. Carney, Growth and effect of mycoplasmas in fallopian tube organ cultures. Br. J. Vener. Dis. 50:212, 1974.
89. Taylor-Robinson, D. Pathogenicity of ureaplasmas for animals and man. Zentralbl. Bakterio. Orig. A. 245:150, 1979.
90. Taylor-Robinson, D., P.M. Furr and A.D.B. Webster, Ureaplasma urealyticum causing persistent urethritis in a patient with hypogammaglobulinaemia. Genitourin. Med. 61:243, 1985.
91. Webster, A.D.B., D. Taylor-Robinson, P.M. Furr, et al., Chronic cystitis and urethritis associated with ureaplasmal and mycoplasmal infection in primary hypogammaglobulinaemia. Br. J. Urol. 54:287, 1982.
92. Bowie, W.R., R.F. Digiacomok, K.K. Holmes, et al., Genital inoculation of male Macaca fascicularis with Neisseria gonorrhoeae and Ureaplasma urealyticum. Br. J. Vener. Dis. 54:235, 1978.
93. Prentice, M.J., D. Taylor-Robinson and G.W. Csonka, Br. J. Vener. Dis. 52:269, 1976.
94. Bowie, W.R., E.R. Alexander, J.F. Floyd, et al., Lancet 2:1276, 1976.
95. Coufalik, E.D.K., D. Taylor-Robinson and C.W. Csonka, Br. J. Vener. Dis. 55:36, 1979.
96. Brown, M.B., G.H. Cassell, D. Taylor-Robinson, et al., J. Clin. Microbiol. 17:288, 1983.
97. Prien, E.L. and C. Frondel, Studies in urolithiasis 1. The composition of urinary calculi. J. Urol. 57:949, 1947.
98. Griffith, D.P. Struvite stones. Kidney Int. 13:372, 1978.
99. Thomsen, A.C. The occurrence of mycoplasmas in the urinary tract of patients with chronic pyelonephritis. Acta. Pathol. Microbiol. Scand. B 83:10, 1975.
100. Thomsen, A.C. Occurrence of mycoplasmas in urinary tract of patients with acute pyelonephritis. J. Clin. Microbiol. 8:84, 1978.
101. Thomsen, A.C. and H.O. Lindskow, Diagnosis of Mycoplasma hominis pyelonephritis by demonstration of urine antibodies. J. Clin. Microbiol. 9:681, 1979.
102. Mardh, P.A. An overview of infectious agents of PID, their biology, and recent advances in methods of detection. Am. J. Obstet. Gynecol. 138:9331, 1980.
103. Wahbeh, C.J., G.B. Hill, R.D. Eden, et al., Intra-amniotic bacterial

colonization in premature labor. Am. J. Obstet. Gynecol., 1984.
104. Bobbit, J.R., C.C. Hayslip and J.D. Damato, Amniotic fluid infection as determined by transabdominal amniocentesis in patients with intact membranes in premature labor. Am. J. Obstet. Gynecol. 140:947, 1981.
105. Cooperman, N.R., M. Kasim and K.R. Rajashekaraiah, Clinical significance of amniotic fluid, amniotic membranes, and endometrial biopsy cultures at the time of cesarean section. Am. J. Obstet. Gynecol. 137:536, 1980.
106. Miller, J.M., M.J. Pupkin and G.B. Hill, Bacterial colonization of amniotic fluid from intact fetal membranes. Am. J. Obstet Gynecol. 136:796, 1980.
107. Bobbitt, J.R. and W.J. Ledger, Amniotic fluid analysis. J. Reprod. Med. 19:8, 1978.
108. Stroup, P.E., Amniotic fluid infection and the intact fetal membrane. Obstet. Gynecol. 19:736, 1962.
109. Caspi, E., F. Solomon, R. Langer, et al., Isolation of mycoplasma from the placenta after cesarean section. Obstet. Gynecol. 48:682, 1976.
110. Gravett, M.G., Causes of preterm delivery. Sem. Perinatol. 8:246, 1984.
111. Goldbus, M.S., W.D. Louhman and C.J. Epstein, Prenatal diagnosis in 3000 amniocenteses. N. Eng. J. Med. 300:157, 1979.
112. The NICHD National Registry for Amniocentesis Study Group: Midtrimester amniocentesis for prenatal diagnosis. Safety and accuracy. J.A.M.A. 236:1471.
113. Milunsky, A. Amniocentesis, genetic disorders and the fetus: Diagnosis, prevention and treatment. A. Milunsky, ed. Plenum, New York, pp. 19-46, 1971.
114. Hanson, F.W., F.R. Tennant, M.Z. Elinor, et al., Analysis of 2136 gentic amniocenteses: Experience of a single physician. Am. J. Obstet. Gyneco. 152:436, 1985.
115. Bartsch, F.K., J. Lundberg and J. Wahlstrom, One thousand consecutive midtrimester amniocenteses. Obstet. Gynecol. 55:305, 1980.
116. Thomsen, A.C., D. Taylor-Robinson, K.B. Hansen, et al., The infrequent occurrence of mycoplasmas in amniotic fluid from women with intact fetal membranes. 63:425, 1984.
117. Schneider, E.L., E.J. Stanbridge and C.J. Epstein, Mycoplasma contamination of cultured amniotic fluid cells: Potential hazard to prenatal chromosomal diagnosis. Science, 184:477, 1974.
118. Weissenbacher, E.R., W. Bredt, W. Jonatha, et al., Utersuchngen Zum Mycoplasmanbefall des Fruchtwasers. Geburtsh U Frauenheilk 36:778, 1976.
119. Platt, R., J.W. Warren and K.C. Edelin. Infection with Mycoplasma hominis in postpartum fever. Lancet 2:1217, 1980.
120. Lamey, J.R., D.A. Eschenbach, L. Tompkins, et al., Isolation of mycoplasmas and bacteria from the blood of postpartum women. Am. J. Obstet. Gynecol. 143:104, 1982.
121. Miller, T.C., S.I. Baman and W.H. Albers, Massive pericardial effusion due to Mycoplasma hominis in a newborn. Am. J. Dis. Child. 136:271, 1982.
122. Dan, M., D.L.J. Tyrrell, G.W. Stemke, et al., Mycoplasma hominis septicemia in a burned infant. J. Pediatr. 99:743, 1981.
123. Baumann, von L. Nachweis von genitalen Mykoplasmen bei kopfschwarteninfektionen von neugeborenen nach interner kardiotokographie. Dt. Gesundh.-Wesen 38:779, 1983.
124. Wallace, R.J., S. Alpert, K. Brown, et al., Isolation of Mycoplasma hominis from blood cultures in patients with postpartum fever. Obstet. Gynecol. 51:181, 1978.

125. Smaron, M.F., S. Boonlayangoor and C.H. Zierdt, Detection of Mycoplasma hominis septicemia by radiometric blood culture. J. Clin. Microbiol. 21:298, 1985.
126. Birch, D.F., K.F. Fairley and R.E. Pavillard, Unconventional bacteria in urinary tract disease: Ureaplasma urealyticum. Kid. Int. 19:58, 1981.
127. Brunner, H., W. Weidner and H.-G. Schiefer, Quantitative studies on the role of Ureaplasma urealyticum in non-gonococcal urethritis and chronic prostatitis. Yale J. Biol. Med. 56:545, 1983.
128. Hofstetter, A. Hautartzt, 28:295, 1977.
129. Gump, D.W., M. Gibson and T. Ashikaga, N. Engl. J. Med. 310:937, 1984.
130. Busolo, F. and R. Zanchetta, The effect of Mycoplasma hominis and Ureaplasma urealyticum on hamster egg in vitro penetration by human spermatozoa. Fertil. Steril. 43:110, 1985.
131. Taylor-Robinson, D. and W.M. McCormack. Mycoplasmas in human genitourinary infections. In the Mycoplasmas. Vol. II. Human and Animal Mycoplasmas. J.G. Tully, R.F. Whitcomb, eds., Academic Press, New York, pp 307-366, 1979.
132. Fodor, M., Differences in the virulence of Ureaplasma urealyticum isolates. Acta. Microbiologica. Sci. Hung. 27:161, 1980.
133. Lamey, J.R., H.M. Foy and G.E. Kenny, Infection with Mycoplasma hominis and T-strains in the female genital tract. Obstet. Gynecol. 44:703, 1974.
134. Sompolinsky, D., F. Solomon, L. Elkina, et al, Infections with mycoplasma and bacteria in induced midtrimester abortion and fetal loss. Am. J. Obstet. Gyneco. 121:610, 1975.
135. Caspi, E., F. Solomon and D. Sompolinsky, Early abortion and Mycoplasma infection. Isr. J. Med. Sci. 8:122, 1972.
136. Stray-Pedersen, B., J. Eng and T.M. Reikvam, Uterine T-mycoplasma colonization in reproductive failure. Am. J. Obstet. Gynecol. 130:307, 1978.
137. Quinn, P.A., A.B. Shewchuk and J. Shuber, et al., Serologic evidence of Ureaplasma urealyticum infection in women with spontaneous pregnancy loss. Am. J. Obstet. Gynecol. 145:245, 1983.
138. Jones, D.M., Br. Med. J. i:338, 1967.
139. Lin, J.-S., K. Radnay, M.I. Kendrick, et al., J. Infect. Dis. 137:266, 1978.
140. Quinn, P.A., A.B. Shewchuck, J. Shuber, et al., Efficacy of antibiotic therapy preventing spontaneous pregnancy loss. Am. J. Obstet. Gynecol. 145:239, 1983.
141. Kundsin, R.B., Mycoplasmas in genitourinary infection and reproductive failure. Prog. Gynecol. 5:275, 1970.
142. Elder, H.A., B.A.G. Santamarina and S. Smith, Am. J. Obstet. Gynecol. 111:441, 1968.
143. Minkoff, H., A.N. Grunebaum, R.H. Schwarz, et al., Risk factors for prematurity and premature rupture of membranes: A prospective study of the vaginal flora in pregnancy. Am. J. Obstet. Gynecol. 150:965, 1984.
144. Lubchenco, L.O., C. Hansman, M. Dressler, et al., Pediatrics 32:793, 1963.
145. Rush, R.W., M.J. Keirse, P. Howat, et al., Contribution of preterm delivery to peinatal mortality. Br. Med. J. 2:965, 1976.
146. O'Brodovich, H.M. and B. Mellins, Bronchopulmonary dysplasia. Am. Rev. Resp. Dis. 132:694, 1985.
147. Maeye, R.L., W.S. Dellinger and W.A. Blanc, J. Pediatr. 79:733, 1971.
148. Tafari, N., S. Ross, R.L. Naeye, et al, Lancet 1:108, 1976.
149. Widmann, F.K., Technical Manual of the American Association of Blood Banks. American Association of Blood Banks, Arlington, V.A. p. 380, 1985.

150. Rudd, P.T., M.B. Brown and G.H. Cassell, A prospective study of Mycoplasma infection in the preterm infant. Isr. J. Med. Sci. 20:899, 1984.
151. Stagno, S., D. Brasfield, M.B. Brown, et al., Infant pneumonitis associated with cytomegalovirus, Chlamydia, Pneumocystis and Ureaplasma; a prospective study. Pediatrics 68:322, 1981.
152. Sherman, M.P., B.W. Goetzman, C.E. Ahlfor, et al., Year Tracheal aspiration and its clinical correlate in the diagnosis of congenital pneumonia. Pediatrics 65:258, 1980.
153. Evans, R.T. and D. Taylor-Robinson, The incidence of tetracycline-resistant strains of Ureaplasma urealyticum. J. Antimicrob. Chemother. 9:1012, 1978.
154. Koutsky, L.A., W.E. Stamm, R.C. Brunham, et al., Persistence of Mycoplasma hominis after therapy: Importance of tetracycline resistance and of coexisting vaginal flora. Sex. Trans. Dis. 10:374, 1983.

*PTR was a Burroughs Welcome Research Fellow from Cambridge University, England and SAH was a visiting scientist from the Wiezmann Institute, Rheovot, Israel. This work was supported by grants HL 19741 and HD 16199 to GHC.

PATHOGENESIS AND MANAGEMENT OF GONORRHEA

Edmund C. Tramont and John W. Boslego

Department of Bacterial Diseases
Division of Communicable Disease and Immunology
Walter Reed Army Institute of Research
Washington, D.C. 20307-5100

Gonorrhea is one of the oldest recorded diseases of mankind (1). Over the past 15 years it has reached epidemic proportions, afflicting principally the most sexually active 15-30 years old age group at a rate of 12/1000/yr. The reasons for such high rates are multifactorial. Increased promiscuity among sexually active adults, the propensity of gonorrhea to remain asymptomatic, the unique epidemiology of the disease and increased antibiotic resistance have all played important roles.

Gonorrhea rates have always been particularly high in the Armed Forces, (2) and presently remain 6 times that of a matched U.S. civilian cohort.

ANTIBIOTIC RESISTANCE

Chromosomally mediated resistance to penicillin has steadily progressed since 1945. Three separate mutations designated Pen A, Pen B, and mtr which are additive have been documented (3,4). The net effect has been that an increasing proportion of strains have become resistant to 2 mcg/ml of penicillin, the in vitro correlate of treatment failure (4). Indeed, the steady increase in resistant strains isolated from the Far East (where historically resistance patterns have changed before those in the U.S.) was documented in 1974 (5). By 1983, treatment failure outbreaks traced to chromosomally mediated resistance had been reported in North Carolina, Tennessee, New Mexico, and Oregon (6). These mutations increase the resistance to penicillin by decreasing the affinity of penicillin binding proteins for beta-lactam antibiotics, by decreasing the permeability of the gonococcal outer membrane, and/or by altering the concentration of penicillin binding proteins (4,7,8).

The first treatment failure due to penicillinase producing N. gonorrhoeae (PPNG) was recorded in 1976 and traced to a contact in the Far East. By 1982, the incidence of PPNG strains in the Far East had skyrocketed to 46% (9). This dictated a change in the treatment-of-choice

"The views of the authors do not purport to reflect the position of the Department of the Army or the Department of Defense," (para 4-3, AR 360-5).

regimen from penicillin to spectinomycin. However, a steady increase in spectinomycin resistant strains has already been reported (9).

Fortunately, a number of newer antibiotics have proved effective for both PPNG and spectinomycin resistant strains (10,11,12). Their principal drawback at this time is cost, a particularly troublesome problem in developing countries.

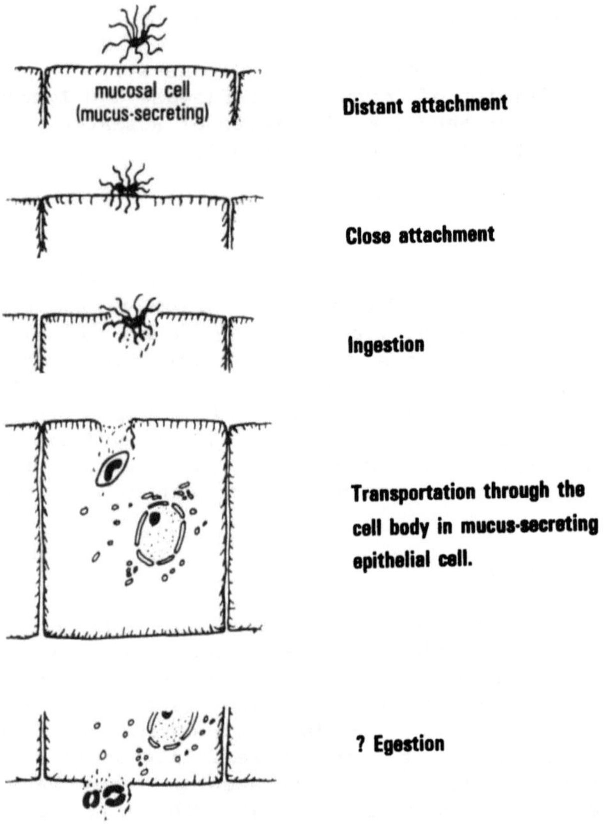


FIGURE 1. THE PATHOGENESIS OF GONOCOCCAL INFECTION

Much has been learned in recent years about the molecular biology of N. gonorrhoeae. The steps in pathogenesis can be broken into 5 stages (1) distant attachment, (2) close attachment (3) ingestion by mucus-secreting cells (4) transportation through the cell body in phagosomes and (5) egestion through the basement membrane (Fig. 1).

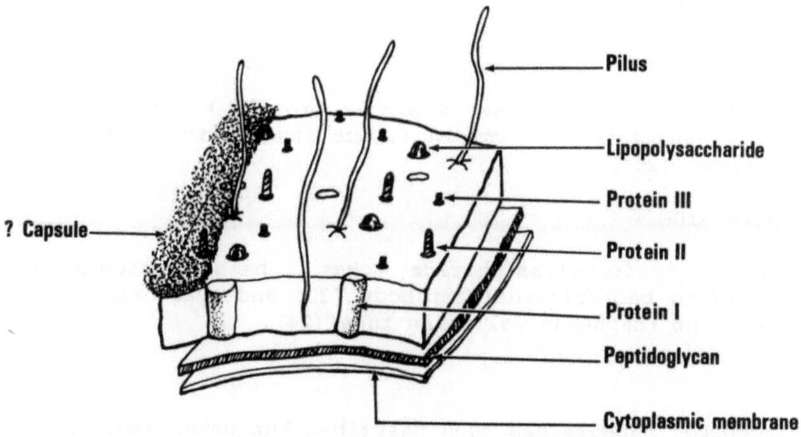


FIGURE 2. SCHEMATIC DIAGRAM OF GONOCOCCAL CELL WALL ADAPTED FROM WHO/VDT/RES/CON/82.137

## PILI

N. gonorrhoeae pili (Fig. 2) are protein organelles of attachment to eukaryotic cells (13,14,15) and they are principally responsible for distant attachment. Antigenically, they consist of a common portion which is shared among all gonococcal pili and a distinct variable portion unique to each strain (16,17,18,19), a situation analogous to the antigenic nature of immunoglobulins. Pili also increase resistance to phagocytosis. A meaningful pilus typing system has not yet been developed.

## PROTEIN I

Protein I functions as a porin, which is a transmembrane channel that permits the exchange of hydrophilic molecules through the hydrophobic outer membrane and is responsible for directly transferring the gonococcus into eukaryotic membranes (20). It has been suggested that they are responsible for increased resistance of gonococci to the lytic activity of normal human sera (21). There are 10-20 known Protein I types.

## PROTEIN II

Protein II is also referred to as the opacity protein because it imparts an opaque quality to colonies grown on modified culture media (22). Opaque colonies tend to be isolated from the male urethra and during the mid-cycle of the menstrual period. Transparent colony types are associated with other phases of the menstrual cycle, fallopian tube and blood isolates. Opaque (O) and transparent (Tr) colony types may or may not be piliated.

## PROTEIN III

All gonococcal strains have a single protein known as Protein III. It is closely associated to Protein I, but its specific role or function is not yet known (20).

## LIPOPOLYSACCHARIDE

Gonococcal lipopolysaccharide has been associated with susceptibility to bacteriocidal antibody (23) and cytotoxic activity for ciliated cells of the human fallopian tube (24).

## CAPSULES

A gonococcal capsule has been described but never isolated (25,26). It has been associated with resistance to phagocytosis (25).

## IgA PROTEASE

Gonococci elaborate an IgA protease which cleaves IgA immunoglobulin at the hinge region (27). The role of IgA protease in infection has not yet been clearly defined.

## IRON BINDING COMPOUNDS

Like most mucosal pathogens, gonococci are efficient scavengers of iron (28). There is evidence that blood and joint isolates, Disseminated Gonococcal Infection (DGI) strains, are more efficient than non-DGI strains (29).

## IMMUNOLOGY

A variety of serological tests that have been developed over the years have repeatedly demonstrated the following: (1) a humoral antibody immunologic response can be invoked by a gonococcal infection, (2) the magnitude and characteristics of the response are not predictable but tend to be more brisk in women, (3) the cross-reactivity with antibody induced by other organisms (natural antibody) is significant and, (4) neither the type or level of antibody correlates with protection.

Local secretory antibody has also been described (30). This antibody functions primarily by blocking the attachment of gonococci to epithelial eukaryotic cells, and this functional aspect of local antibody is directed principally at pili (31). This antibody is broadly cross-reactive against heterologous strains (30-32).

Repeated gonococcal infections are common suggesting that immunity does not exist. However, Mahoney, et al. (33) demonstrated relative resistance to infection which correlated with a history of previous gonococcal infections (older prostitutes have fewer episodes of symptomatic gonorrhea), and Brinto, et al. have demonstrated significant protection in a human challenge model (34).

Nevertheless, there are many factors which appear to mediate against effective immunity to gonorrhea. Immunity may be strain specific and the heterogenicity of pili and cell membrane Protein I or Protein II may thus mediate against the development of broad resistance. Immunity may be easily overwhelmed. Local antibody, which principally acts by directly blocking the attachment of gonococci to mucosal cells, lacks the augmentation and efficiency supplemented by complement (bacteriocidal or opsonic antibodies). Thus, a small number of organisms can overwhelm the host's immune status. Indeed, Brinton, et al. found that increasing the concentration of organisms from $10^3$ to $10^5$ organisms increased infectivity from $\leq 10\%$ to $\geq 90\%$ in a human challenge model (34).

## CLINICAL SYNDROMES

**Urethritis and Cervicitis.** Urethritis and cervicitis are the most common clinical presentations of gonorrhea. In contrast to long held views, gonococcal cervicitis is symptomatic in about 50% of cases. The reasons for this misconception stems from the earlier descriptions of patients referred to sexually transmitted disease clinics as contacts, the failure to culture urine of high risk patients on appropriate culture media and the nonspecific nature of the complaints. The complaints, which range from lower abdomen pain, urgency, frequency and vaginal discharge, are most prominent at the time of menses and are often disregarded as dysmenorrhea.

**Pelvic Inflammatory Disease (PID).** Women bear a disproportionate amount of the morbidity due to sexually transmitted disease. The incidence of PID and ectopic pregnancy is increasing. At least 40% of cases of PID are due to gonorrhea. Once PID occurs, the individual is at greater risk of suffering a second episode. Infertility increases with each episode (35), and by the time the patient has suffered her sixth episode of PID, she has a 95% chance of being sterile.

A strategy to protect against the development of PID with a Protein I vaccine has been proposed and is undergoing phase I trials (Buchanan, T., personal communication).

**Epididymitis.** Epididymitis is the male equivalent of PID. Today, chlamydia causes epididymitis among young sexually active men more often then *N. gonorrhoeae* (36).

*Asymptomatic Carriage*. Asymptomatic carriage occurs most often in women, although 10-15% of men are also asymptomatic. However, a careful history will often elicit the presence of a slight discharge ("do you stain your underwear?"), abdominal discomfort or urinary tract symptoms.

*Oropharyngitis*. Approximately 5% of all individuals who report to a STD clinic with gonorrhea have gonococcal pharyngitis manifested by a severe sore throat. Oral-genital sex is the most frequent antecedent history. The clinical microbiology laboratory must be advised to plant the throat specimen on selective media. A Gram stain revealing intracellular Gram negative diplococci is very suggestive (in the appropriate setting). Oropharyngitis is an important consideration affecting antibiotic treatment (see below).

*Conjunctivitis*. Gonococcal conjunctivitis may be a consequence whenever a fetus passes through an infected or colonized birth canal. The incidence of neonatal conjunctivitis decreased significantly after the institution of silver nitrate eye drops. Adults may also develop conjunctivitis. (*N. gonorrhoeae*, like most genital tract pathogens, have a tropism for the conjunctiva and the oropharynx).

*Proctitis*. Gonococcal proctitis, a potential consequence of anal sex, often presents with a discharge, tenesmus or rectal abcess.

*Disseminated Gonococcal Infection (DGI)*. DGI occurs most often in women, especially during menses and late pregnancy. It has been speculated that these strains have an increased capacity to utilize free iron, and therefore behave in a more virulent fashion (29). DGI strains in this country tend to be of an $A^-H^-U^-$ auxotype, quite sensitive to penicillin (37,38) and resistant to the lytic activity of normal serum (39,40).

Tenosynovitis and septic arthritis are the most common complications of DGI. Endocarditis and meningitis are quite rare. Most patients present with fever and migratory synovitis which finally "settles" in one joint. The knee and elbow are the most frequently involved joints. Skin lesions, which range from tiny macula to discrete pustules, characteristically develop on the ankles, feet, wrist, hands and fingers.

## DIAGNOSIS

The Gram stain and culture remain the most reliable methods to diagnose gonorrhea. The Gram stain is 93-99% specific for gonococcal urethritis or cervicitis. It is 93% sensitive in men but only 60% sensitive in women. Therefore, one should always perform a Gram stain on specimens obtained from both sexes, but a negative Gram stain in a women requires a culture before assigning an alternative diagnosis.

Culture on selective media remains the most sensitive means of diagnosis in women. As noted above, urine cultures on selective media for N. *gonorrhoeae* are under used! (*N. gonorrhoeae* is an important etiologic agent causing the urethral frequency syndrome and urine cultures on selective media for *N. gonorrhoeae* should be done on all sexually active populations.)

A number of newer techniques utilizing monoclonal antibodies and DNA hybridization have recently been introduced. To date, they are not superior to the Gram stain or culture, but offer hope for a quicker diagnosis in women by eliminating the 24-48 hr delay for culture results.

## TREATMENT

Penicillin remains the treatment of choice for uncomplicated gonorrhea in the United States (1984) (Table 1) (4). How long this will

TABLE 1. Treatment of Uncomplicated Gonorrhea

| |
|---|
| Aqueous procaine penicillin G (APPG), 4.8 m units IM plus 1.0 gm Probenicid PO[1,2] |
| or |
| Amoxicillin, 3.0 gm plus 1.0 gm Probenicid PO[1] |
| or |
| Ampicillin, 3.5 gm plus 1.0 gm Probenicid PO[1] |
| or |
| Spectinomycin, 2.0 gm IM[1] |

[1]Plus doxycycline 100 mg PO bid or tetracycline 500 mg PO qid X 7 days.
[2]Recommended for homosexual men and pharyngeal infections.

remain the case is conjecture. Penicillin cannot be used in patients who have contracted their illness in the Far East. Spectinomycin is the drug of choice for patients infected with PPNG strains but the rapid increase in spectinomycin resistance is troublesome. Ampicillin 3.5 gm or Amoxicillin 3.0 gm given orally with 1 gm of probenecid can be substituted for penicillin. Because at least 40% of patients have a concomitant chlamydia infection, the addition of a tetracycline antibiotic is important, especially when the ability to verify the diagnosis of chlamydia is poor or lacking. Doxycycline 100 mg bid or tetracylcine 0.5 gm qid for 7 days is usually adequate (42).

Patients with DGI should be hospitalized to rule out endocarditis, meningitis, and optimally manage septic joints. Since patients with disseminated gonococcal infection are usually infected with strains that are quite sensitive to penicillin, hospitalization for 3 days of intravenous penicillin is usually adequate to cure the infection (37). Furthermore, surgical drainage of infected joints is not necessary.

Patients with gonococcal oropharyngitis are more difficult to treat, and may require more then one course of treatment. Spectinomycin is not reliable as treatment for pharyngeal gonorrhea (43).

Since pelvic inflammatory disease is so frequently a mixed infection and the possible consequence is so devastating, antimicrobial combinations to cover N. gonorrhoeae, anaerobic bacteria, enterobacteriaceae and C. trachomatis are warranted (Table 2). PPNG strains may be treated with a variety of newer antibiotics (Table 3).

TABLE 2. Treatment of Pelvic Inflammatory Disease

| Anaerobic Coverage | | | Daily Dose |
|---|---|---|---|
| Cefoxitin | IM or IV | | 2.0-8.0 gm |
| Metronidazole | PO or IM or IV | | 1.0-2.0 gm |
| Enterobacteriaceae | | | |
| Cefoxitin | IM or IV | | 2.0-8.0 gm |
| 3rd generation cephalosporin[2] | | IM or IV | |
| Aminoglycoside | IM or IV[2] | | |
| Chlamydia | | | |
| Doxycycline | PO or IV[3] | | 100-200 mg |

[1]The length of treatment depends upon severity of disease. Most often 10-14 days of treatment is sufficient. Toxic patients should be admitted to the hospital.
[1]Daily dose depends on drug chosen and renal status.
[3]14 days of treatment.

**TABLE 3. Treatment PPNG (Anywhere where incidence is greater than 1%)**

| |
|---|
| Spectinomycin, 2.0 gm. IM |
| or |
| Cefoxitin, 2.0 gm. IM |
| or |
| Cefotaxime, 1.0 gm. IM plus 1.0 gm probenicid PO |
| or |
| Ceftriaxone, 250 mg. IM |
| or |
| Norfloxacin, 1200 mg. PO |

## REFERENCES


1. Preuss, J. Biblical and Talmudic Medicine (1911). F. Rosner (trans). New York. Sand hedrin Press, (1978).
2. Roseburg, T. Microbes and Morals. The Strange Story of Venereal Diseases. New York. The Viking Pess, (1971).
3. Jaffe, H.W., A.L. Schroeter, G.H. Reynolds, A.A. Zaidi, J.E. Martin and J.D. Thayer. Pharmacokinetic determinants of penicillin cure of gonococcal urethritis. Antimicrob. Ag. & Chemother. 15:587, (1979).
4. Martin, J.E., A. Lester, E.V. Price and J.D. Schamle. Comparative study of gonococcal susceptibility to penicillin in the United States, 1955-1969. J. Infect. Dis. 122:459, (1970).
5. Wilson, C., D.L. Rose and E.C. Tramont. Increased antibiotic resistance of Neisseria gonorrhoeae in Korea. Antimicrob. Ag. & Chemother. 9:716, (1976).
6. Chromosomally mediated resistant Neisseria gonorrhoeae - United States. Morbid. Mortal. Week. Rep. 33:408, (1984).
7. Sparling, P.F., F.A. Sarubbi, Jr., and E. Blackman. Inheritance of low-level resistance to penicillin, tetracycline, and chloramphenicol in: Neisseria gonorrhoeae. J. Bacteriol. 124:740, (1975).
8. Dougherty, T.J., A. Koller and A. Thomasz. Penicillin binding proteins of penicillin susceptible and intrinsically resistant Neisseria gonorrhoeae. Antimicrob. Ag. Chemother. 18:730, (1980).
9. Piziak, M.V., C. Woodbury, D. Berliner, E. Takafuji, J. Kirkpatrick, S. Opal and E. Tramont. Resistance trends of Neisseria gonorrheae in the Republic of Korea. Antimicrob. Ag. & Chemo. 25:7, (1984).
10. Berg, S.W., M.E. Kilpatrick, W.O. Harrison and J.A. McCutchan. Cefoxitin as a single-dose treatment for urethritis caused by penicillinase-producing Neisseria gonorrhoeae. N. Engl. J. Med. 300:509, (1979).
11. Ng, W.S., D.V. Chau, J. Ling, P. Echeverria, R. Rockhill and K. Arnold. Penicillinase producing N. gonorrhoeae isolates from S.E. Asia. Brit. J. Vener. Dis. 59:232, (1983).
12. Crider, S.R., S.D. Colby, L.K. Miller, W.O. Harrison, S.B.J. Kerbs and S.W. Berg. Treatment of penicillin-resistant Neisseria gonorrhoeae with oral norfloxacin. N. Eng. J. Med. 311:137, (1984).
13. Swanson, J.S., S.J. Kraus and E.C. Gotschlich. Studies on gonococcus infection. I. Pili and zones of adhesion: their relation to gonococcal growth patterns. J. Exp. Med. 134:886, (1971).
14. Swanson, J. Studies of gonococcal infection. IV. Pili: their role in attachment of gonococci to tissue culture cells. J. Exp. Med. 137:571, (1973).
15. Pearce, W.A. and T. Buchanan. Attachment role of gonococcal pili. J. Clin. Invest. 61:931, (1978).

16. Schoolnik, G.K., R. Fernandez, J.Y. Tai, J. Rothbard and E.C. Gotschlich. Gonococcal pili, primary structure and receptor binding domain. J. Exp. Med. 159:1351, (1984).
17. Rothbard, J.B., R. Fernandez and G.K. Schoolnik. Strain-specific and common epitopes of gonococcal pili. J. Exp. Med. 160:208, (1984).
18. Boslego, J.W., R. Chung, D.M. McChesney, J. Ciak, J.S. Sadoff, M. Piziak, J. Brown, E. Tramont, C. Brinton, S. Wood and J. Bryan. Efficacy trial of a parenteral gonococcal pilus vaccine. Submitted for publication, (1985).
19. Tramont, E.C., J.W. Boslego, R. Chung, D.M. Chesney, J. Ciak, J. Sadoff, M. Piziak, C. Brinton, S. Wood and J. Bryan. Parenteral gonococcal pilus vaccines in pathogenesis of pathogenic Neisseria, ed G Schoolnik, Am. So. Microbiol. Washington, D.C. To be published.
20. Blake, M.S. and E.C. Gotschlich. Gonococcal membrane proteins: speculation on their role in pathogenesis. Prog. Allergy 33:258, (1983).
21. Hook, E.W., III, D.A. Olsen and T.M. Buchanan. Analysis of the antigen specificity of the human serum immunoglobulin G immune response to complicated gonococcal infection. Infect. Immun. 43:706, (1984).
22. Hechels, J.E. The surface properties of N. gonorrhoeae: isolation of the major components of the outer membrane. J. Gen. Micro. 99:333, (1977).
23. Tramont, E.C., J.C. Sadoff and C. Wilson. Variability of the lytic susceptibility of N. gonorrhoeae to human sera. J. Immun. 118:1843, (1977).
24. McGee, Z.A., A.P. Johnson and D. Taylor-Robinson. Pathogenic mechanisms of N. gonorrhoeae: observations on damage to human fallopian tubes in organ culture by gonococci of colony type 1 or type 4. J. Infect. Dis. 143:413, (1981).
25. Richardson, W.P. and J.C. Sadoff. Production of a capsule by Neisseria gonorrhoeae. Infect. Immun. 15:663, (1977).
26. Hendley, J.O., K.R. Powell, N.L. Salomonsky and R.R. Rodewald. Electron microscopy of the gonococcal capsule. J. Infect. Dis. 143:796, (1981).
27. Plaut, A.G., J.V. Gilbert, M.S. Artenstein and J.D. Capra. Neisseria gonorrhoeae and Neisseria meningitis: extracellular enzyme cleaves human immunoglobulin A. Science. 190:1103, (1975).
28. Mickelson, P.A. and P.F. Sparling. Ability of N. gonorrhoeae, N. meningitis and commensal Neisseria species to obtain iron from transferrin and iron compounds. Infect. Immun. 33:555, (1981).
29. Payne, S.M., K.K. Holmes and R.A. Finkelstein. Role of iron in disseminated gonococcal infections. Infect. Immun. 20:573, (1978).
30. Tramont, E.C. and J. Ciak. Antigonococcal antibodies in genital secretions, in: Immunobiology of Neisseria gonorrhoeae, Am. Soc. Microbiol., pp 174-276, (1978).
31. Tramont, E.C. Inhibition of adherence of Neisseria gonorrhoeae by genital secretions. J. Clin. Invest. 59:117, (1977).
32. Tramont, E.C., J.W. Boslego, R. Chung, D. McChesney, J. Ciak, J. Sadoff, M. Piziak and C.C. Brinton. Gonococcal pilus vaccine in bacterial vaccines. J. Robbins ed., Thieme-Stratton, Inc., (1985).
33. Mahoney, J.F., C. Ferguson and M. Bucholtz. The use of penicillin sodium in the treatment of sulfonamide-resistant gonorrhea in men. Am. J. Syph. Gonorr. Vener. Dis. 27:525, (1943).
34. Brinton, C.C., Jr., S.W. Wood, A. Brown, A.M. Labik, J.R. Lee, S.W. Polen, E.C. Tramont, J.C. Sadoff and W.D. Zollinger. The development of a neisserial pilus vaccine for gonorrhea and meningococcal meningitis, in: Reviews Inf. Dis. International Symposium on Bacterial Vaccines, pg. 140, ed. Robbins, Hill, Sadoff. Thieme-Stratton, Inc., New York, (1982).

35. Westrom, L. Incidence, prevalence and trends of acute pelvic inflammatory disease and its consequence in industrialized countries. Am. J. Obs. and Gyn. 138:880, (1980).
36. Berger, R.E., R.E. Alexander, G. Monda, J. Ansell, G. McCormick and K.K. Holmes. Chlamydia trachomatis as a cause of acute idiopathic epididymitis. N. Eng. J. Med. 298, (1978).
37. Wiesner, P.H., H.H. Handsfield and K.K. Holmes. Low antibiotic resistance of gonococci causing disseminated infection. N. Engl. J. Med. 288:1221, (1973).
38. Knapp, J.S. and K.K. Holmes. Disseminated gonococcal infection caused by Neisseria gonorrhoeae with unique nutritional requirements. J. Infect. Dis. 132:204, (1975).
39. Tramont, E.C., J.C. Sadoff and C. Wilson. Variability of the lytic susceptibility of Neisseria gonorrhoeae to human sera. J. Immunol. 118:1843, (1977).
40. Schoolnik, G.K., T.M. Buchanan and K.K. Holmes. Gonococci causing disseminated gonococcal infection are resistant to the bactericidal action of normal human sera. J. Clin. Invest. 58:1163, (1976).
41. Sexually transmitted diseases treatment guidelines 1982. Morbid. Mortal. Week. Rep. (Suppl). 31:35, (1982).
42. Stamm, W.E., M.E. Guinan, C. Johnson, S. Sturcher, K.K. Holmes and W.M. McGormack. Effect of treatment regimens for Neisseria gonorrhoeae on simultaneous infections with Chlamydia trachomatis. N. Engl. J. Med. 310:545, (1984).
43. Schroeter, A.L., G.H. Reynolds, K.K. Holmes, T. Pyke and P.J. Wiesner. Spectinomycin in the treatment of gonorrhea. J. Am. Vener. Dis. Ass. 1:139, (1975).

# NEW DEVELOPMENTS IN THE ETIOLOGY AND PATHOGENESIS OF BACTERIAL VAGINOSIS

Carol A. Spiegel

Director of Clinical Microbiology
University of Wisconsin Hospital and Clinics
Madison, Wisconsin 53791-9452

## INTRODUCTION

Vaginitis by definition means inflammation of the vagina and is to be distinguished from cervicitis which has its own set of pathogens. We are aware of relatively few agents that cause vaginitis. *Trichomonas vaginalis*, a protozoan parasite, is usually associated with a voluminous, often frothy, green vaginal discharge. Yeast vaginitis is usually caused by the yeast-like fungus *Candida albicans* and is characterized by a curd-like vaginal discharge often associated with itching. Vaginitis caused by these two agents has been termed specific vaginitis and represents approximately 50% of all cases. Patients presenting to a physician with complaints of vaginitis but having evidence of neither *T. vaginalis* nor *C. albicans* were defined as having nonspecific vaginitis (NSV). NSV is not a new syndrome. As early as 1895, Kronig (1) published drawings of vaginal fluid from patients with NSV which showed a mixed flora devoid of large rods and including vibrio-like organisms. Later Doderlein (cited in reference 2) described three grades of vaginal flora. Grade I, defined as a clean vagina, contained large rod-shaped organisms which became known as Doderlein's bacilli and represent various species of the genus *Lactobacillus*. Grade II was a mixed flora, and Grade III, the pathological flora, was notable by its absence of the large rod-shaped organisms. Kronig's drawings and Doderlein's description of the Grade III flora are characteristic of the syndrome we now call NSV.

The vaginal discharge associated with *T. vaginalis* and *C. albicans* is usually characterized by a large number of white blood cells. In contrast, few white cells are seen in vaginal fluid from patients with NSV. The term vaginosis connotes increased fluid flow from the vagina but does not imply an increase in the number of white blood cells. Because this syndrome is associated with bacteria rather than protozoa or fungi, we have suggested that the term bacterial vaginosis (BV) be used (3).

## CLINICAL CRITERIA

The criteria used in the clinical diagnosis of BV were originally described by Gardner and Dukes (4), refined by Pheifer et al. (5), and verified by Amsel et al. (6). The presence of three of the four following signs is consistent with a diagnosis of BV; 1) a homogeneous, white, adherent vaginal discharge, 2) vaginal fluid pH greater than 4.5, 3) a fishy odor on addition of potassium hydroxide, and 4) the presence of clue cells, vaginal epithelial cells coated with coccobacillary organisms.

## Gardnerella vaginalis

In 1953 Leopold (7) and in 1955 Gardner and Dukes (4) described a small coccobacillary organism which was associated with BV. Gardner and Dukes named the organism Haemophilus vaginalis. Because the organism requires neither X (hemin) nor V (NAD) factors, it cannot be placed in the genus Haemophilus. Based on its Gram stain morphology, the organism was then placed in the genus Corynebacterium and was named C. vaginale. However, because it lacks the enzyme, catalase, and does not have arabinose in its cell wall, it could not remain in that genus. Further taxonomic studies have shown that this organism does not resemble any previously described genus and has since been named Gardnerella vaginalis (8,9). Because Gardner and Dukes isolated G. vaginalis from 92% of women with a clinical diagnosis of BV and from no control patients, they concluded that it was the etiologic agent of BV. Subsequent studies by others were not able to reproduce those findings. For instance, McCormick et al. (10) isolated G. vaginalis from 38% of patients with BV and 30% of controls. Some of these discrepancies were due to the use of nonstandard methods for the clinical diagnosis of BV. For instance, some authors diagnosed BV by exclusion (symptoms in the absence of T. vaginalis or C. albicans) rather than on the presence of three out of the four signs mentioned above. Other discrepancies were due to the use of various methods for culture and identification of G. vaginalis.

G. vaginalis is a relatively fastidious organism which requires a complex medium, carbon dioxide, and humidity for optimum growth. In 1980, Totten et al. (11) developed a selective differential medium for isolation of G. vaginalis from vaginal fluid. The medium is called human blood bilayer tween (HBT) agar. It contains colistin and nalidixic acid to inhibit facultative Gram-negative rods such as E. coli, amphotericin B to inhibit yeast, and a thin agar layer containing human blood cells to optimize the hemolytic activity of G. vaginalis. G. vaginalis is the only gram-positive, rod-shaped organism which is $\beta$-hemolytic on this medium when it is incubated in an atmosphere containing 5% carbon dioxide. Using HBT, the authors showed that while nearly 100% of patients with BV were vaginally colonized by G. vaginalis, as many as 69% of patients without BV also had G. vaginalis in their vaginal fluid. Therefore, this organism is part of the endogenous vaginal flora. While 91% of BV patients and 26% of controls had 3 to 4 + G. vaginalis in their vaginal fluid, the predictive value of a positive culture with 3 to 4 + G. vaginalis was only 49%. The predictive value of a negative test was 97%.

## Amines

Another characteristic of BV is the fishy odor which can be detected either by addition of potassium hydroxide in vitro or semen in vivo. Chen et al. (12,13) have determined that this odor is due to the presence of amines, the decarboxylation products of amino acid metabolism. Cadaverine and putrescine, the decarboxylation products of lysine and arginine, respectfully, are the two predominant amines in vaginal fluid of patients with BV. These compounds are not produced by G. vaginalis, but they are produced by the mixed aerobic and anaerobic flora recovered from patients with BV.

## Anaerobic Bacteria

Pheifer et al. (5) noted an increase in the prevalence of anaerobic bacteria in BV. They also noted that patients responded to therapy with metronidazole, an antimicrobial agent with activity against anaerobic but not aerobic bacteria. Subsequent studies have shown an increase in both the prevalence and quantity of certain anaerobic organisms, such as Bacteroides bivius, B. disiens, B. melaninogenicus, Peptostreptococcus, Peptococcus, Eubacterium, and curved rods (14,15,16).

## Laboratory Diagnosis of Bacterial Vaginosis

The major change in vaginal flora from a) lactobacilli with or without G. vaginalis to b) a mixture of anaerobic bacteria and G. vaginalis in the absence of lactobacilli can be detected by two methods: gas-liquid chromatography (14) and direct Gram stain (17) of vaginal fluid. Gas-liquid chromatography is used to identify the by-products of carbohydrate and protein metabolism by bacteria. Lactobacilli produce lactic acid, Bacteroides produce succinic acid, Gardnerella produces acetic acid, peptostreptococci produce acetic acid with or without butyric acid, and the vaginal curved rods produce succinic and acetic acids. Therefore, as one would predict, GLC analysis shows that normal vaginal fluid contains a large amount of lactic acid but little of the other acids, while vaginal fluid from patients with BV contains less lactic acid and increased succinic and acetic acids. Direct Gram stain of vaginal fluid from a control patient reveals large gram positive bacilli of the Lactobacillus morphotype, with or without small gram-variable bacilli of the Gardnerella morphotype. Direct Gram stain of vaginal fluid from a BV patient reveals little or no Lactobacillus morphotype and large numbers of organisms resembling Gardnerella, Bacterioides, anaerobic cocci, and curved rods.

## Mobiluncus Species

Vaginal curved rods were detected in vaginal fluid before the turn of the century (1), but documentation of their association with BV awaited the 1980's (16,18,19). The first strain was isolated by Curtis in 1913 (20) from a patient with postpartum endometritis. Five additional strains were characterized by Moore in 1954 (21). In 1980, Durieux and Dublanchet (22) characterized 18 additional strains and were the first to suggest the presence of two types which were distinguishable by cell size, carbohydrate utilization, and susceptibility to metronidazole. Other workers found from one to three types (23,24,25). While the characteristics examined, methods used, and results reported varied considerably from one publication to the next, all studies agreed that these anaerobic rods were motile and produced succinic acid. Further examination of their phenotypic and genotypic characteristics revealed that these organisms were not related to any known genus of anaerobic bacteria and so were placed in a new genus, Mobiluncus, which means "motile hooks" (26). The genus name Falcivibrio has also been suggested for these organisms (27). Mobiluncus species are susceptible to penicillin, ampicillin, clindamycin and vancomycin, and are resistent to colistin and nalidixic acid (22,24). This susceptibility pattern is typical of Gram-positive organisms, however, Mobiluncus species are Gram-variable. Electron microscopic characterization of their cell walls reveals a morphology not consistent with either a typical Gram-negative or Gram-positive cell (26,27). The genus Mobiluncus is divided into two species. M. curtisii are small (1.7 um) cells which often stain Gram-positive. Mobiluncus mulieris are larger cells (2.9 um) which usually stain Gram-negative. These two species can be distinguished from one another by biochemical tests. M. curtisii can be further divided into two subspecies (26).

The susceptibility of these organisms to metronidazole, the drug of choice for treating BV, is of interest. Skarin et al. (24) have reported that all strains of organisms consistent with M. mulieris are susceptible to metronidazole, while all strains with a morphology consistent with M. curtisii are resistent to metronidazole. We have found that all strains of M. curtisii are resistent to metronidazole, but we have also found some resistent strains of M. mulieris (Speigel, unpublished data). Approximately 12% of BV patients treated with an adequate dose of metronidazole will have persistent or recurrent disease within four weeks after therapy (28). The role of metronidazole-resistant strains of Mobiluncus in treatment failures is unknown.

## Pathogenesis

There are very few studies on the role of any of these organisms in the pathogenesis of BV. Piot et al. (29) recently developed a biotyping scheme for strains of G. vaginalis. Using tests for lipase activity, β-galactosidase, and hippurate hydrolysis, they found 1) the same three biotypes predominated in the United States of America, Belgium and Zaire, 2) the vaginal biotypes remained consistent for a one week period; 3) the same biotype was found in the urethra of male sexual partners of women with BV if they were cultured within 24 hours of sexual contact; and 4) no specific biotype was associated with BV. These data suggest that G. vaginalis is a sexually transmitted organism, but the biotyping scheme was unable to incriminate particular strains as agents of BV.

Other studies of pathogenesis have focused on hemagglutination by Mobiluncus species (30) and, pH dependence of attachment of vaginal anaerobic organisms to epithelial cells (31,32) and human erythrocytes (14). There have also been some attempts at development of animal models (34,35). Most data, however, on the pathogenesis of bacterial vaginosis are derived from the response of patients to therapy with various antimicrobial agents, most notably ampicillin, amoxicillin or metronidazole (28).

Ampicillin and amoxicillin are β-lactam antibiotics which have activity against G. vaginalis in vitro. Isolates of B. bivius from the upper female genital tract have been shown to possess β-lactamase and so are not inhibited by these drugs (36). If vaginal isolates of these organisms also possess β-lactamase, we would predict that the drug would be inactivated in vivo and so would inhibit neither the Bacteroides nor the Gardnerella. Clinically this appears to be the case. Within 7 to 14 days of beginning therapy with ampicillin or amoxicillin, 57% of patients have persistent or recurrent BV. As many as 44% of patients continue to have clue cells, 30% have an abnormal discharge, 83% have a vaginal pH greater than 4.7, 22% have a positive KOH odor test, 56% have biochemical evidence of the presence of abnormal amines, 39% have an abnormal GLC and up to 76% have 3 to 4 + G. vaginalis in their vaginal fluid.

Metronidazole is a nitroimidazole antimicrobial agent with activity against anaerobic bacteria and the anaerobic protozoa Giardia lamblia and T. vaginalis. Four weeks after initiation of therapy with metronidazole, 12% of patients had recurrent or persistent BV (28). Seven to 14 days after onset of therapy, no patient had clue cells, 11% had an abnormal discharge, 58% had a pH greater than 4.7, 5% had a positive amine odor test, 5% had biochemical evidence of amines, none had an abnormal GLC, and 5% had 3 to 4 + G. vaginalis.

Although the parent compound of metronidazole is not active against G. vaginalis in vitro, Ralph and Amatnieks (37) have shown that the hydroxymetabolite of metronidazole does have activity against G. vaginalis in vitro. They used these data to explain why this drug eliminates G. vaginalis from the vagina. Another possible explanation is that during BV, products of metabolism by the anaerobic bacteria stimulate the growth of G. vaginalis. When the anaerobes are inhibited by metronidazole and their products are no longer available, the number of G. vaginalis may fall below detectable levels or it may be totally eliminated from the vagina. Clarification of the actual role of metronidazole in eliminating G. vaginalis from the vagina awaits further investigation.

The effect of antimicrobial therapy on vaginal lactobacilli also adds insight to the pathogenesis of this infection. Persistent and recurrent BV occurs more commonly after treatment with ampicillin or amoxicillin than after treatment with metronidazole, a drug which is inactive against lactobacilli. If lactobacilli facilitate the return of a normal vaginal ecosystem by lowering the vaginal pH and thereby making the oxidation-reduction potential less conducive for growth of anaerobic organisms, we would expect better regrowth of lactobacilli in patients treated with metronidazole than those treated with ampicillin or amoxicillin. We have tested this hypothesis in two ways (28). We have used direct Gram stain of vaginal fluid as a method to monitor recolonization by lactobacilli following therapy. One or more large Lactobacilli morphotypes were seen in each oil immersion field from nine of nine patients treated with metronidazole and only one of 10 patients treated with ampicillin or amoxicillin. Seven of the 10 patients treated with ampicillin or amoxicillin had no detectable Lactobacillus morphotype on direct Gram stain. Second, we used GLC to look for a change in the concentration of lactic acid in vaginal fluid after therapy. While the average increase in the lactic acid peak height was 29 mm following therapy with ampicillin, it was 113 mm following therapy with metronidazole. Both of these pieces of data suggest that metronidazole more readily allows recolonization of the vagina by lactobacilli.

SUMMARY

Bacterial vaginosis is unlike the "classic" sexually transmitted diseases. Unlike cervical infection with Chlamydia or salpingitis caused by N. gonorrhoeae, no single etiologic agent has been identified, and the organisms which are associated with infection have all been found as members of endogenous vaginal flora, with the possible exception of Mobiluncus species. If, as we suspect, BV is due to interactions among various organisms found in the vagina during vaginal health, we must determine what changes in the microbial or chemical ecology determine the development of BV. If, for instance, BV is simply due to an inversion in the concentrations of various organisms such that the anaerobes which are usually present in low numbers become predominant and the lactobacilli which usually predominate become few in number, we must determine which causes what. That is, does some organism or environmental change allow the anaerobes to overgrow and thereby inhibit the lactobacilli, or does some change inhibit the lactobacilli, thereby, allowing the other flora to overgrow? Answers to questions such as these await further research.

REFERENCES

1. I. Kronig. Uber die Natur der Scheidenheme, Speciell uber das vorkommen anaerorber Streptokokken in Scheidensekret Schwangerer. Centralbl. fur Gynakol. 19, 409, (1895).

2. R. Cruickshank, and A. Sharman. The biology of the vagina in the human subject. J. Obstet. Gynecol. Br. Emp. 41, 208, (1934).
3. K.K. Holmes, C. Spiegel, R. Amsel, D.A. Eschenbach, K.C.S. Chen, and P. Totten. Nonspecific vaginosis. Scand. J. Infect. Dis. Suppl. 26, 110, (1981).
4. H.L. Gardner, and C.D. Dukes Hemophilus vaginalis vaginitis. Am. J. Obstet. Gynecol. 69, 962, (1955).
5. T.A. Pheifer, P.S. Forsyth, M.A. Durfee, H.M. Pollock, and K.K. Holmes. Nonspecific vaginitis: Role of Haemophilus vaginalis and treatment with metronidazole. N. Engl. J. Med. 298, 1429, (1978).
6. R. Amsel, P.A. Totten, C.A. Spiegel, K.C.S. Chen, D. Eschenbach, and K.K. Holmes. Nonspecific vaginitis: Diagnostic criteria and microbial and epidemiologic associations. Am. J. Med. 74, 14, (1983).
7. S. Leopold. Heretofore undescribed organism isolated from genitourinary system. U.S. Armed Forces Med. J. 4, 263, (1953).
8. P. Piot, E. Van Dyck, M. Goodfellow, and S. Falkow. A taxonomic study of Gardnerella vaginalis (Haemophilus vaginalis) Gardner and Dukes. J. Gen. Microbiol. 119, 373, (1980).
9. J.R. Greenwood, and M.J. Pickett. Transfer of Haemophilus vaginalis Gardner and Dukes to a new genus, Gardnerella (Gardner and Dukes) comb. nov. Int. J. Syst. Bacteriol. 30, 170, (1980).
10. W.M. McCormack, C.H. Hayes, B. Rosner, J.R. Evrard, V.A Crockett, S. Alpert, and S.H. Zinner. Vaginal colonization with Corynebacterium vaginale (Haemophilus vaginalis). J. Infect. Dis. 136, 740, (1977).
11. P.A. Totten, R. Amsel, J. Hale, P. Piot, and K.K. Holmes. Selective differential human blood bilayer media for isolation of Gardnerella (Haemophilus) vaginalis. J. Clin. Microbiol. 15, 141, (1982).
12. K.C.S. Chen, P.S. Forsyth, T.M. Buchanan, and K.K. Holmes. Biochemical aspects of nonspecific vaginitis: Amine content of vaginal fluid from untreated patients. J. Clin. Invest. 63, 828, (1979).
13. K.C.S. Chen, R. Amsel, D.A. Eschenbach, and K.K. Holmes. Biochemical diagnosis of vaginitis: Determination of diamines in vaginal fluid. J. Infect. Dis. 145, 337, (1982).
14. C.A. Spiegel, R. Amsel, D. Eschenbach, F. Schoenknecht, and K.K. Holmes. Anaerobic bacteria in nonspecific vaginitis. N. Engl. J. Med. 303, 601, (1980).
15. E. Taylor, A.L. Blackwell, D. Barlow, and I. Phillips. Gardnerella vaginalis, anaerobes, and vaginal discharge. Lancet. i, 1376, (1982).
16. A.L. Blackwell, A.R. Fox, I. Phillips, and D. Barlow. Anaerobic vaginosis (non-specific vaginitis): Clinical, microbiological, and therapeutic findings. Lancet. ii, 1379, (1983).
17. C.A. Spiegel, R. Amsel, and K.K. Holmes. Diagnosis of bacterial vaginosis by direct Gram stain of vaginal fluid. J. Clin. Microbiol. 18, 170, (1983).
18. C.A. Spiegel, D.A. Eschenbach, R. Amsel, and K.K. Holmes. Curved anaerobic bacteria in bacterial (nonspecific) vaginosis and their response to antimicrobial therapy. J. Infect. Dis. 148, 817, (1983).
19. J.L. Thomason, P.C. Schreckenberger, W.N. Spellacy, L.J. Riff, and L.J. LeBeau. Clinical and microbiological characterization of patients with nonspecific vaginosis associated with motile, curved anaerobic rods. J. Infect. Dis. 149, 801, (1984).
20. A.H. Curtis. A motile curved anaerobic bacillus in uterine discharges. J. Infect. Dis. 12, 165, (1913).
21. B. Moore. Observations on a group of anaerobic vaginal vibrios. J. Path. Bact. 67, 461, (1954).
22. R. Durieux, and A. Dublanchet. Les "Vibrions" anerobies des leucorrhees. Technique d'isolement et sensibilite aux

antibiotiques. Med. Mal. Infect. 10, 109, (1980).
23. C. Pahlson, V. Forsum, A. Hallen, E. Hjelm, and J. Wallin. Characterization of motile anaerobic curved rods isolated from women with lower genital tract infection in three different countries. Eur. J. Sex. Trans. Dis. 1, 73, (1983).
24. A. Skarin, E. Holst, and P.-A. Mardh. Antimicrobial susceptibility of comma-shaped bacteria isolated from the vagina. Scand. J. Infect. Dis. Suppl. 40, 81, (1983).
25. M.S. Sprott, H.R. Ingham, R.S. Pattman, R.L. Eisenstadt, G.R. Short, H.K. Narang, P.R. Sisson, and J.B. Selkon. Characteristics of motile curved rods in vaginal secretions. J. Med. Microbiol. 16, 175, (1983).
26. C.A. Spiegel, and M. Roberts, Mobiluncus gen. nov., Mobiluncus curtisii subspecies curtisii sp. nov., Mobiluncus curtisii subspecies holmesii subsp. nov., and Mobiluncus mulieris sp. nov., curved rods from the human vagina. Int. J. System Bacteriol. 34, 177, (1984).
27. R. Hammann, A. Kronibus, A. Viebahn, and H. Brandis, Falcivibrio grandis gen. nov. sp. nov. and Falcivibrio vaginalis gen. nov. sp. nov., a new genus and species to accommodate anaerobic motile curved rods formerly described as "Vibrio mulieris" (Prevot 1940) Breed et al. 1948. System Appl. Microbiol. 5, 81, (1984).
28. R. Amsel, C.W. Critchlow, C.A. Spiegel, K.C.S. Chen, D. Eschenbach, K. Smith, and K.K. Holmes. Comparison of metronidazole, ampicillin, and amoxicillin for treatment of bacterial vaginosis (nonspecific vaginitis): Possible explanation for the greater efficacy of metronidazole. In U.S. Metronidazole Conference, Proceedings from a Symposium, (S.M. Finegold ed.), p. 225. Biomedical Information Corporation, New York, (1982).
29. P. Piot, E. Van Dyck, M. Peeters, J. Hale, P.A. Totten, and K.K. Holmes. Biotypes of Gardnerella vaginalis. J. Clin. Microbiol. 20, 677, (1984).
30. P.-A. Mardh, and S. Svensson. Hemagglutination by vaginal anaerobic curved rods and its inhibition by oligosaccharides. In Bacterial vaginosis, (P.-A. Mardh and D. Taylor-Robinson ed.)., Almqvist & Wiskell International, Stockholm, 179, (1984).
31. B. Fredericsson, A.-K. Moller, and C.E. Nord. Can Gardnerella vaginalis and anaerobic curved rods attach to vaginal epithelial cells in vitro, resulting in clue cells. In Bacterial vaginosis, (P.-A. Mardh and D. Taylor-Robinson ed.), Almqvist & Wiskell International, Stockholm, 195, (1984).
32. H. Moi, D. Danielsson, and F. Schoenknecht. An in vitro study of the attachment to vaginal epithelial cells and anaerobic curved rods, Bacteriodes bivius and Bacterioides disiens. In Bacterial vaginosis, (P.-A. Mardh and D. Taylor-Robinson ed.), Almqvist & Wiskell International, Stockholm, 185, (1984).
33. C.A. Ison, and C.S.F. Easmon. Studies on the mechanism of adhesion of Gardnerella vaginalis to human erythrocytes. In Bacterial vaginosis, (P.-A., Mardh and D. Taylor-Robinson ed.), Almqvist & Wiskell International, Stockholm, 191, (1984).
34. A.P. Johnson, C.A. Ison, C.M. Hetherington, M.F. Osborn, G. Southerton, W.T. London, C.S.F. Easmon, and D. Taylor-Robinson. Vaginal colonization of pig-tailed macaques by Gardnerella vaginalis. In Bacterial vaginosis, (P.-A. Mardh and D. Taylor-Robinson ed). Almqvist & Wiskell International, Stockholm, 207, (1984).
35. P.-A. Mardh, E. Holst, and B.R. Moller. The grivet monkey as a model for study of vaginitis. Challenge with anaerobic curved rods and Gardnerella vaginalis. In Bacterial vaginosis, (P.-A. Mardh and D. Taylor-Robinson ed.). Almqvist & Wiskell International, Stockholm, 201, (1984).

36. C.E. Nord, and B. Olsson-Liljequist. Resistance to -lactam antibiotics in Bacteroides species. J. Antimicrob. Chemother. 8 Suppl. D, 33, 1981.
37. E.D. Ralph, and Y.E. Amatnieks. Relative susceptibilities of Gardnerella vaginalis (Haemophilus vaginalis), Neisseria gonorrhoeae, and Bacteroides fragilis to metronidazole and its two major metabolites. Sex. Trans. Dis. 7, 157, 1980.

# NONRADIOACTIVE DNA HYBRIDIZATION: APPLICATION TO CLINICAL MICROBIOLOGY

Norman Kelker, Majorie Pollice and Huey-Lang Yang

Enzo Biochem, Inc.
325 Hudson Street
New York, NY 10013

## INTRODUCTION

While nucleic acid hybridization has been used to great benefit by molecular biologists, the application to clinical use has been limited. This is due to the requirement to label probe DNA with phosphorus-32 ($^{32}P$). Since this isotope has a short half-life (14.1 days) and emits a high energy beta particle, $^{32}P$-labeled probes are short-lived and require special handling conditions and licensing. The recent development of nonradioactive DNA labeling procedures (1) presents the opportunity to apply the benefits of nucleic acid hybridization to routine clinical use. Diagnostic procedures based on this technology are being developed for clinical microbiology.

## DNA HYBRIDIZATION

Nucleic acid hybridization, developed by Marmur et al. (2), detects nucleotide sequences by the matching of complementary strands. In practice, one DNA sample, the target, is immobilized on a solid support such as a nitrocellulose membrane or a glass slide or coverslip. The other DNA sample, the probe, is labeled. Radioactive labeling most commonly uses $^{32}P$, although $^{3}H$ (tritium) is better suited to some procedures. The nonradioactive procedure, described below, uses biotin convalently attached to either deoxyuridine triphosphate (Bio-11-dUTP, Fig. 1) or to deoxycytidine triphosphate (Bio-11-dCTP). Denatured, immobilized target DNA and labeled, denatured, soluble probe DNA are mixed and incubated under conditions favorable to renaturation. Excess probe is washed away and the hybrization of complementary sequences between the two samples is determined by the presence of label on the solid support.

Nucleic acid hybridization offers several advantages to clinical microbiology use. The specificity inherent in the nucleotide sequence is extremely favorable. For example, the probability of the occurence of a sequence in nucleotides in length is $1/4^n$. Thus, a sequence of only 13 nucleotidies would appear on the average of once in every $4^{13}$ or 67,108,864 nucelotides, a length which exceeds the genome complexity of most microbial pathogens. This example must be qualified since partially homologous sequences such as those which differ in only one or two nucleotides, or those which are completely homologous to a continuous sequence of, for example, 11 of the 13 nucleotides of the target sequence would also hybridize. However, gene cloning procedures can be applied to isolate those sequences which are specific and do not crosshybridize organisms.

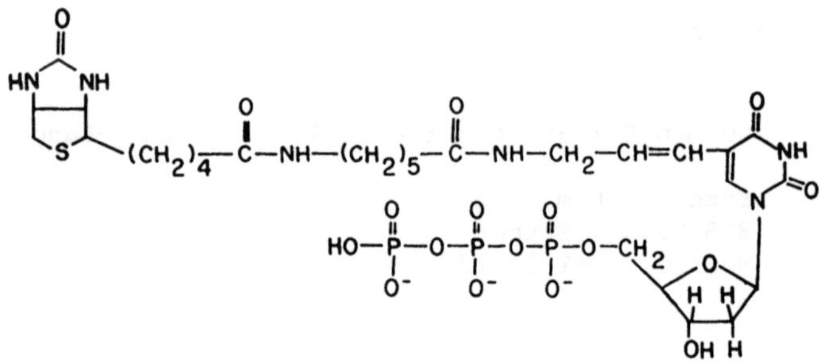

Figure 1.

Bio-11-dUTP substitutes for thymidine triphosphate in nick translation Biotin-reactions. (2'-DEOXYURIDINE TRIPHOSPHATE 5-ALLYLAMINE-BIOTIN).

DNA is stable and can withstand harsh treatment. Boiling and strong aklali treatment are, in fact, standard DNA denaturation procedures. Unlike most proteins, DNA is stable to formaldehyde. Thus, conditions for transport and storage of clinical samples can be greatly simplified.

DNA hybridization can be done very rapidly. Hybridization kinetics have been characterized by Wetmur and Davidson (3). Since the DNA concentration determines the frequency of intermolecular collisions, the rate of reassociation of complementary sequences (hybridization) can be increased by increasing the DNA concentration. Thus, the use of high probe concentration can reduce the hybridization time required to yield a visible signal to a few minutes.

## NONRADIOACTIVE PROCEDURES FOR DNA LABELING AND DETECTION

The development of nonradioactive DNA labeling procedures by Langer, Waldrip and Ward (1), offers the opportunity to apply the advantages of nucleic acid hybridization procedures to routine clinical use. In this procedure, a nonradioactive moiety, the reported molecular, is covalently bound to DNA in a way which does not disrupt normal helix formation. This is done by the substitution of a biotinylated nucleotide, Bio-11-dUTP (Fig. 1), for thymidine monophosphate residues in the DNA probe by a nick translation reaction (4). The attachment of biotin, through an 11 atom linker arm, to position 5 in the pyrimidine ring does

Not interfere with helix formation. Hybridization rates for DNA substituted with Bio-11-dUTP and for unsubsTituted DNA are identical (1,5). Therefore, biotinylated DNA probes can be used in established hybridization protocols.

Visualization of biotinylated, hybridized probe DNA is done by procedures based on the recognition of biotin. Biotin-binding proteins such as avidin, streptavidin or antibiotin antibodies are used with fluorescent dyes, such as fluorescein and rhodamine, or color-producing enzymes, such as horseradish peroxidase, alkaline phosphatase or acid phosphatase.

Complexes of streptavidin with biotinylated enzymes are especially useful. These multienzyme complexes are constructed by mixing a multiply biotinylated enzyme molecule and either streptavidin or avidin, both of which have four biotin binding sites. Since there are unoccupied biotin binding sites in the multienzyme complex, it will bind to biotinylated DNA. AFter removal of excess unbound complex, a substrate is added which, together with a chromogen, yields a colored product. A schematic representation of the hybridization/detection procedure is shown in Fig. 2.

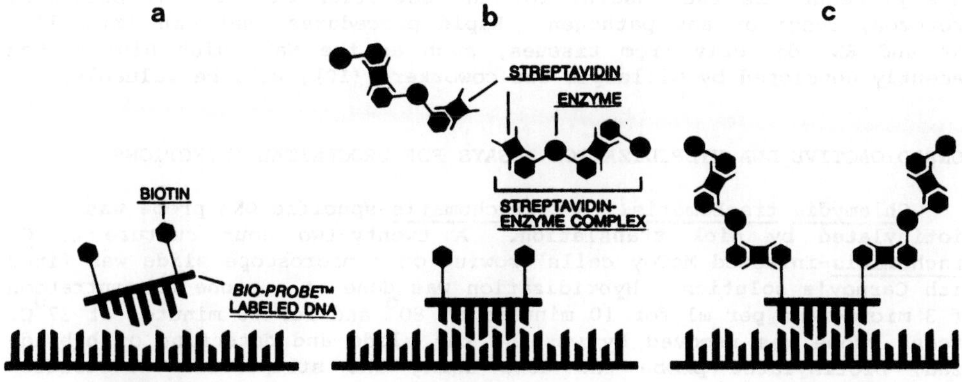


Figure 2.

A. Nonradioactive hybridization/detection procedures. Visualization is done by the addition of substrate and chromogen to yield a colored product.

a - Hybridization; b = Addition of detection complex; c = Detection.

Substrates and chromogens can be chosen to meet the needs of the assay. Assays which require high resolution, such as localization of target sequences to a cell nucleus or to a band on a southern blot, require a substrate which yields an insoluble, visible precipitate. The horseradish peroxidase chromogen, diaminobenzidine, which, together with $_2O_2$, yields a brown precipitate, is extremely useful in this regard. The alkaline phosphatase substrate 5-bromo-4-chloro 3-indolyl phosphate together with nitroblue tetrazolium is also excellent. Furthermore, substrates which yield a variety of colors are available. A large variety of substrates which yield soluble, colored products is available.

## FORMATS FOR DETECTION OF PATHOGENS

A number of hybridization procedures, e.g., Southern blotting (6), Northern blotting (7), colony hybridization (8,13) and in situ hybridization (9), have been developed to meet specific needs. All are fully compatible with nonradioactive DNA hybridization. While all of these techniques may be useful to varying degrees in clinical microbiology, the most likely procedures to gain widespread use will be those in which DNA from clinical samples can be directly and rapidly fixed on a solid support, i.e., in situ and dot blot hybridizations. In this way, direct assay of the clinical sample without the requirement for culture and isolation procedures, i.e., "no growth" assays, can be developed.

In situ hybridization procedures are especially useful for detection of viruses and other intracellular patogens, e.g., *Chlamydia trachomatis*. Cells present in a clinical sample, such as a tissue scrape for genital herpes, are fixed on a glass slide or coverslip and hybridization and detection procedures are done. In dot blot hybridization, DNA (or RNA) from a clinical sample is fixed directly in a small area, usually less than 2 mm in diameter, onto nitrocellulose or other suitable membranes. This procedure is thus useful for the detection of viruses, bacteria, protozoa, fungi or any pathogen. Rapid procedures that can immobilize DNA and RNA directly from tissues, such as the NaI Quick Blot method recently developed by Gillespie and coworkers (10), will be valuable.

## NONRADIOACTIVE DNA HYBRIDIZATION ASSAYS FOR UROGENITAL INFECTIONS

*Chlamydia trachomatis*. A *C.trachomatis*-specific DNA probe was biotinylated by nick translation. A twenty-two hour culture of *C. trachomatis*-infected McCoy cells growing on a microscope slide was fixed with Carnoy's solution. Hybridization was done at a probe concentration of 3 micrograms per ml for 10 minutes at $80^{o}$ and for 60 minutes at $37^{o}C$. Excess probe was removed by washing the slide and detection of hybridized, biotinylated probe was done using the streptavidin-horseradish peroxidase complex (DETEK 1-hrp, Enzo Biochem). Visualization was achieved by the addition of $H_2O_2$ and the chromogen diaminobenzidine.

Infected cells appear as obvious darkened cytoplasmic inclusions (Fig. 3). Thirteen serotypes of *C. trachomatis* have been tested and all give a positive signal in this test.

Ampicillin resistance: Resistence to ampicillin results from a plasmid mediated beta-lactamase which is encoded in a tranposon structure, TnA (11). Homologous TnA sequences appear in *Haemophilus influenzae*, *E. coli* and *Neisseria gonorrhoeae*. Nonradioactive colony hybridization procedures were applied to clinical isolates of N. gonorrhoeae growing as isolated colonies on chocolate agar. The colonies were transferred to cellulose paper (Whatman 541) by pressing the sterile membrane onto the agar surface. DNA hybridization was done using as probe a Col El derived plasmid which carries TnA (12). The probe was biotin-labeled by nick translation. The colony hybridization procedure was done by a modification of the Taub and Thompson procedure (13) and detection was done using DETEK 1-hrp. Ampicillin resistant colonies appear as dark spots on the nitrocellulose membrane (Fig. 4).

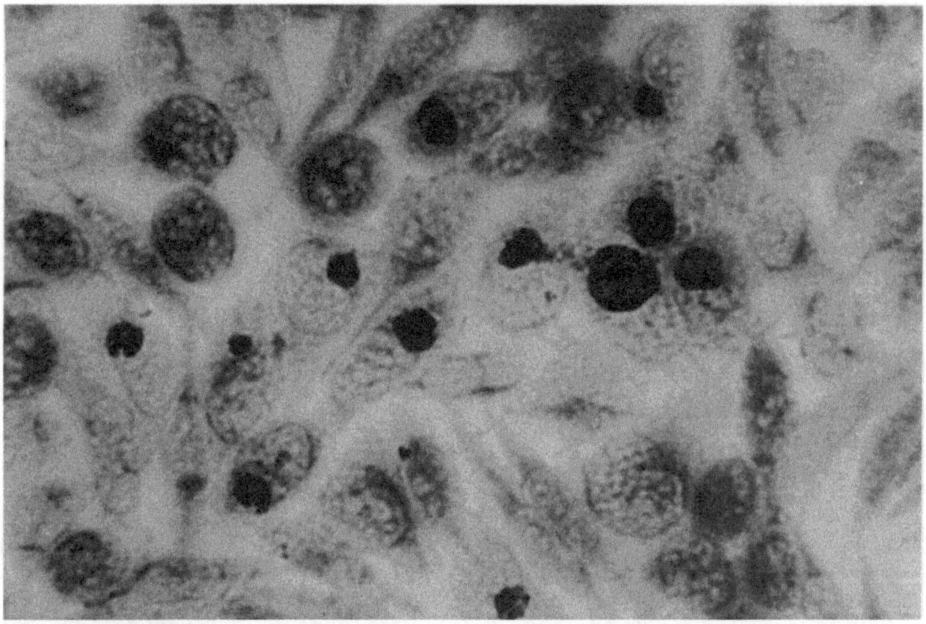

Figure 3.

Chlamydia trachomatis detection in infected McCoy cells. Chlamydia appears as dark cytoplasmic inclusions. Both infected and uninfected cells can be seen.

DISCUSSION

DNA hybridization procedures offer an exciting approach to clinical diagnosis of microbial pathogens. In addition to the studies reported here, work is underway in several laboratories to take advantage of the nonradioactive technology (14,15,16). The format that reaches the clinical laboratory will be the one that meets the requirements for user friendliness, reliability and speed. Clearly DNA hybridization procedures can be developed to meet these needs.

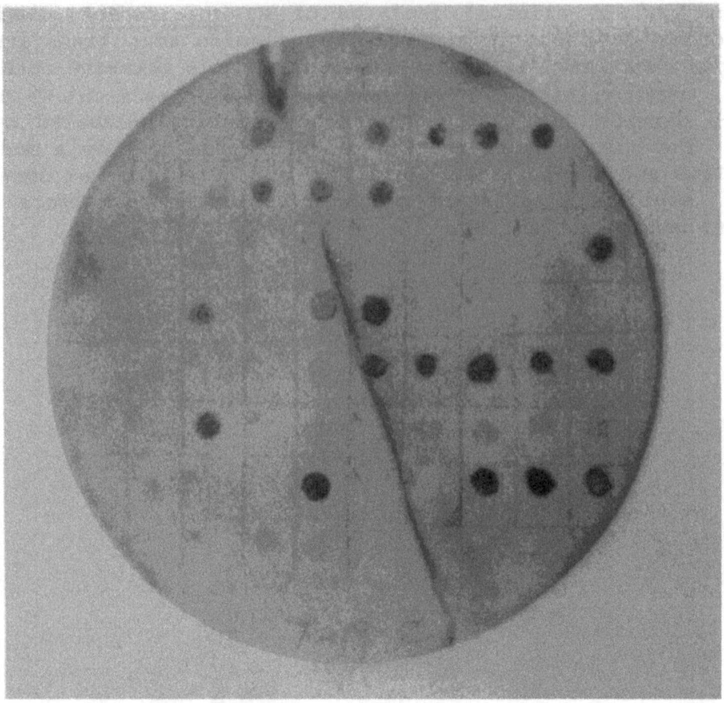

Figure 4.

Detection of ampicillin resistance in clinical samples of Neisseria gonorrhoeae by colony hybridization procedures.

REFERENCES


1. Lnager, P.R., A.A. Waldrop and D.C. Ward. Enzymatic synthesis of biotin-labeled polynucleotides: Novel nucleic acid affinity probes. Proc. Natl. Acad. Sci. USA. 78: 6633, (1984).
2. Marmur, J., R. Rownd and C.L. Schildkraut. Denaturation and renaturation of deoxyribonucleic acid, Prog. Nucleic Acids Res. 1: 231, (1963).
3. Wetmur, J. and N. Davidson. Kinetics of renaturation of DNA. J. Mol. Biol. 31: 349, 1968.
4. Rigby, P.W.J., M. Dieckmann, C. Rhodes and P. Berg. Labelling deoxyribonucleic acid to high specific activity in vitro by nick translation with DNA polymerase I, J. Mol. Biol. 113: 237, (1977).
5. Gardner, L. Non-radioactive DNA labeling: detection of specific DNA and RNA sequences on nitrocellulose and in situ hybridization, Biotechniques 1: 38, (1983).
6. Southern, E.M. Detection of specific sequences among DNA fragments separated by gel electrophoresis, J. Mol. Biol. 98: 503, (1975).
7. Alwine, J.C., D.J. Kemp and G.R. Stark. Methods for detection of specific RNA's in agarose gels by transfer to diazobenzyloxymethyl paper and hybridization with DNA probes, Proc. Natl. Acad. Sci. USA 74: 5350, (1977).

8. Grunstein, M. and D. Hogness. Colony hybridization: a method for the isolation of cloned DNA's that contain a specific gene, Proc. Natl. Acad. Sci. USA 72: 3961, (1975).
9. Gall, J. and M.L. Pardue. Nucleic acid hybridization in cytological preparations, Methods Enzymol. 21: 470, (1971).
10. Gillespie, D. and J. Bresser. mRNA Immunobilization in NaI: Quick-blots, Biotechniques, 1: 184, (1983).
11. Heffron, F., C. Rubens and S. Falkow. Transporttion of a plasmid DNA sequence which mediates ampicillin resistance: general description and epidemiologic considerations, in DNA Insertion Elements, Plasmids and Epsisomes, Bakhari, Shapiro and Adhya, eds. Cold Spring Harbor, New York (1977).
12. Inselburg, J. Isolation, mapping and examination of effects of TnA insertions in Col E1 plasmids, J. Bacteriol. 129: 482, (1977).
13. Taub, F. and E.B. Thompson. An improved method of preparing large arrays of bacterial colonies containing plasmids for hybridization: In situ purification and stable binding of DNA on paper filters. Analyt. Biochem. 126: 222, (1982).
14. Sixbey, J.W., E.H. Vesterinen, J.G. Nedrud, N. Raab-Traub, L.A. Walton and J.S. Pagano. Replication of Epstein-Barr virus in human epithelial cells infected in vitro, Nature. 306: 480, (1983).
15. Sixbey, J.W., J.G. Nedrud, N. Raub-Traub, R.A. Hanes and J.S. Pagano. Epstein-Barr virus replication in oropharyngeal epithelial cells, N. Engl. J. Med. 310: 1225 (1984).
16. Brigati, D.J., D. Myerson, J.J. Leary, B. Spanholz, S.Z. Travis, C.K.Y. Frong, G.D. Hsiung and D.C. Ward. Detection of viral genomes in cultured cells and paraffin-embedded tissue sections using biotin-labeled hybridization probes, Virology, 126: 32, (1983).

PARTICIPANTS

P. Weiner, M.D. and D. Kaye, M.D.
Department of Medicine
The Medical College of Pennsylvania
Philadelphia, Pennsylvania 19129

Richard C. Tilton, Ph.D.
Professor of Laboratory Medicine
University of Connecticut Health Center
Farmington, Connecticut 06032

S. Grant Mulholland, M.D. and Kenneth Weisman, M.D.
Department of Urology
Jefferson Medical College
Philadelphia, Pennsylvania 19107

Prabhavathi B. Fernandez, Nathan L. Shipkowitz, and Robert R. Bower
Pharmaceutical Products Division
Abbott Laboratories
North Chicago, Illinois

Gary K. Schoolnik, M.D., Peter O'Hanley, M.D., Ph.D., David Lark, M.D., Staffan Normark, M.D., Kenneth Vosti, M.D., and Stanley Falkow, Ph.D.
Medical Service, Palo Alto Veterans Administration Medical Center
and The Departments of Medicine and Medical Microbiology
Stanford University School of Medicine
Stanford, California

Julius Schachter, Ph.D.
University of California, San Francisco
Building 30, Room 416
1001 Potrero Avenue
San Francisco, California 94110

Michale R. Spence, M.D., M.P.H., and Joan F. Adler, M.D.
Department of Obstetrics and Gynecology
Hahnemann University School of Medicine
Philadelphia, Pennsylvania 19102

Ruth B. Kundsin, Sc.D.
Brigham and Women's Hospital
Department of Microbiology and Molecular Genetics
Harvard Medical School
Boston, Massachusetts 02115

G.H. Cassell[1], J.K. Davis[2], K.B. Waites[1,3], P.T. Rudd[1], D. Talkingon[1], D. Crouse[4], and S.A. Horowitz[1]
[1]Department of Microbiology
[2]Department of Comparative Medicine
[3]Department of Pathology and Spain Rehabilitation Center
[4]Department of Pediatrics
University of Alabama Schools of Medicine and Dentistry
Universityof Alabama at Birmingham
University Station
Birmingham, Alabama 35294

Edmund C. Tramont and John W. Boslego
Department of Bacterial Diseases
Division of Communicable Disease and Immunology
Walter Reed Army Institute of Research
Washington, D.C. 20307-5100

Carol A. Speigel, Ph.D.
Director of Clinical Microbiology
University of Wisconsin Hospital and Clinics
Madison, Wisconsin 53791-9452

Norman Kelker, Majorie Pollice, and Huey-Lang Yang
Enzo Biochem, Inc.
325 Hudson Street
New York, New York 10013

Alan T. Evangelisa, Ph.D.
Microbiology Department
Cooper Hospital/University Medical Center
Camden, New Jersey 08103

INDEX

MIX
Papier aus verantwortungsvollen Quellen
Paper from responsible sources
FSC® C105338

If you have any concerns about our products,
you can contact us on
**ProductSafety@springernature.com**

In case Publisher is established outside the EU,
the EU authorized representative is:
**Springer Nature Customer Service Center GmbH**
**Europaplatz 3, 69115 Heidelberg, Germany**

Printed by Libri Plureos GmbH
in Hamburg, Germany